An Atlas of Tumours
Involving the
Central Nervous System

An Atlas of Tumours Involving the Central Nervous System

ROBIN O. BARNARD

Neuropathologist, The National Hospitals for
Nervous Diseases, Maida Vale, London

VALENTINE LOGUE

Professor of Neurosurgery
Department of Neurosurgical Studies
Institute of Neurology, Queen Square, London

&

PATTERSON S. REAVES

Neurosurgeon, Baylor University Medical Center, Dallas, Texas

with a foreword by
LUCIEN J. RUBINSTEIN

Professor of Pathology (Neuropathology)
Stanford University School of Medicine

BAILLIÈRE · TINDALL

LONDON

BAILLIÈRE TINDALL
7 & 8 Henrietta Street, London WC2E 8QE

Cassell & Collier Macmillan Publishers Ltd, London
35 Red Lion Square, London WC1R 4SG
Sydney, Auckland, Toronto, Johannesburg

The Macmillan Publishing Company Inc.
New York

First published 1976

ISBN 0 7020 0465 0

Published in the United States of America by
The Williams and Wilkins Company, Baltimore

Printed by The Whitefriars Press Ltd, London and Tonbridge

CONTENTS

Contents

FOREWORD

The last few years have witnessed a resurgence of interest in neuro-oncology. Much of it is due to the discovery of new potent neuro-oncogenic agents and the exploitation of sophisticated laboratory techniques, many of which are now providing biomedical investigators with a growing body of data. New tools are being devised for the experimental study of brain tumours utilizing radiotherapeutic, chemotherapeutic and immunological methods. The prospects for neuro-oncological research in the next decade are likely to be rewarding.

Meanwhile the classical information accumulated in the past fifty years on the biology and morphology of human cerebral tumours remains the cornerstone upon which the complex edifice of neuro-oncological research must be constructed, and, for each new generation of students, the need continues for this knowledge to be passed on clearly, systematically and accurately. The present monograph fills this need. It is the fruit of the harmonious collaboration of a neuropathologist and two neurosurgeons. The authors have opted to present their subject by juxtaposing a carefully selected collection of coloured photomicrographs with a sampling of illustrative clinical and neurosurgical diagnostic problems based on actual case histories. In one volume the features of a systematic atlas and those of a series of succinct cliniconeuropathological case descriptions are therefore amalgamated; such a desirable blend of clinical and microscopical information is not usually available in the more conventional atlas or textbook of neuropathology or in current treatises of neurosurgery. The authors' concrete approach will hold much attraction for the budding neurosurgeon on his first exposure to neuropathology, for the junior pathologist confronted at the beginning of his career by the somewhat bewildering variety of neurosurgical diagnostic problems, for the senior medical student embarking on his neurology or neurosurgery clerkship, and for the preceptor of medicine who wishes to establish a meaningful correlation between the clinical and the morphological aspects of human brain tumours in the course of his teaching. For the post-doctoral as well as for the medical student in need of a rapid review, the text and illustrations will provide a clear synoptic account of a rather complex subject. Every medical reader will surely gain from such a felicitous partnership of two neurological disciplines. We have here a concise and lucid presentation of correlative neuropathology that is worthy of every success.

August 1975

LUCIEN J. RUBINSTEIN, M.D.
Professor of Pathology (Neuropathology),
Stanford University School of Medicine,
Stanford, California.

vii

PREFACE

The management of patients with intracranial and intraspinal neoplasms makes up a large part of the practice of every neurologist and neurosurgeon. And for appropriate management, accurate diagnosis is essential. In recent years, the use of radioactive isotopes and improved radiological methods, including the E.M.I. scanner, have contributed much towards recognition and localization of tumours, but ultimately diagnosis must rest upon the microscopical examination of tissue removed at operation. Thus knowledge of the appearances presented by different tumours, and some understanding of the difficulties which may be encountered in the interpretation of these appearances, are of crucial importance both for the pathologist who examines the tissue, and for the clinician upon whose judgement the patient depends.

The problems inherent in the accurate diagnosis of biopsy specimens of brain tumours are seldom discussed in textbooks. Indeed, a superficial examination of well-known works of reference may well lead the inexperienced either to the opinion that immediate classification of any tumour is possible on the basis of the examination of a few cells, or that the whole subject is so confusing that it cannot be mastered and, like a magic art, must be left in the hands of a few skilled interpreters.

There is a need, therefore, for a book that is sufficiently elementary to make no great demands upon the reader's existing knowledge of neuropathology, but which illustrates clearly some of the patterns of appearance typical of the tumours that commonly occur, and of those of less common occurrence that often raise special problems. There is no doubt that the most satisfactory way to gain experience in making diagnoses is to take a box of slides, a microscope, and some notes of the clinical presentation of each case. In this book we have attempted to provide something on these lines: a brief history of the patient's illness, enough to focus attention on the diagnostic possibilities, followed by a more detailed pathological description, together with coloured illustrations as a substitute for the microscope. It is possible, thus, for the reader to make a clinical, and then a pathological, diagnosis for each case; and to associate the particular pattern of each tumour with details of a particular patient.

To emphasize this association, other aspects have received less attention. There are no pictures of the naked-eye appearance of tumours; no illustrations of radiological findings; and little attention is paid to special pathological methods such as metallic impregnations, to histochemistry or to electronmicroscopy. In the choice of material no attempt has been made to be comprehensive; rather, it is hoped, that by being selective it will be possible to show where some of the special difficulties lie, and also to provide an essential background of experience to make further progress in understanding the subject more rapid and more easy.

The authors are indebted to the members of the staff of the National Hospitals for Nervous Diseases for their cooperation, and would especially like to thank Mr Lindsay Symon, several of whose cases figure in this book. Professor Lucien J. Rubinstein has generously written our foreword and has criticized our typescript: we are grateful for his constructive comments and also for providing the transparencies reproduced as Figs 1 and 2 on Plate 19. Our thanks go to Dr J. E. Olvera Rabiela for the slide reproduced as Fig. 4 on Plate 19, and to Dr H. Pambakian for Fig. 2 on Plate 59.

The skilled technical work of several of the staff of the laboratory at Maida Vale Hospital is the basis for the illustrations in this Atlas, and we would like to express our appreciation to them all. The majority of the photomicrographs were taken by Mr Trevor Scott whose high standards it is a pleasure to acknowledge. For secretarial assistance our thanks go to Mrs F. M. Hall.

The photomicrographs illustrated in this volume were taken on a Zeiss photomicroscope using Kodachrome II A film.

ROBIN O. BARNARD
VALENTINE LOGUE
PATTERSON S. REAVES

August 1975

GENERAL BIBLIOGRAPHY

A list of references will be found at the end of each section of the book, augmented by a small bibliography consisting of articles that the authors can recommend. Each selection is an arbitrary one.

BAILEY, P., BUCHANAN, D. N. and BUCY, P. C. (1939) *Intracranial Tumors of Infancy and Childhood.* Chicago: University of Chicago Press.

BAILEY, P. and CUSHING, H. (1926) *A Classification of Tumors of the Glioma Group.* Philadelphia: Lippincott (An important, and justly famous, landmark).

BLACKWOOD, W., DODDS, T. C. and SOMMERVILLE, J. C. (1964) *Atlas of Neuropathology.* Edinburgh and London: E. & S. Livingstone (37 pages with 54 illustrations are devoted to tumours).

MCMENEMEY, W. H. (1966) In *Systemic Pathology,* ed. G. Payling Wright and W. St C. Symmers, vol. 2. London: Longmans.

MINCKLER, J. (1971) *Pathology of The Nervous System,* vol. 2. New York: McGraw-Hill (Over 300 pages deal with the pathology of tumours: various authors).

POON, T. P., HIRANO, A. and ZIMMERMAN, H. M. (1971) *Electron Microscopic Atlas of Brain Tumors.* New York and London: Grune & Stratton.

RUBINSTEIN, L. J. (1972) *Tumors of the Central Nervous System. Atlas of Tumor Pathology,* Second Series, Fascicle 6. Washington: Armed Forces Institute of Pathology (Both an atlas and a textbook).

RUSSELL, DOROTHY S. and RUBINSTEIN, L. J. (1971) *Pathology of Tumours of the Nervous System,* 3rd ed. London: Arnold (Regarded widely as the authoritative text).

SLOOFF, J. L., KERNOHAN, J. W. and MACCARTY, C. S. (1964) *Primary Intramedullary Tumors of the Spinal Cord and Filum Terminale.* Philadelphia: Saunders (Data on 301 cases).

VINKEN, P. J. and BRUYN, G. W. (1974) *Handbook of Clinical Neurology: Tumours of the Brain and Skull,* vol. 16, 17, 18. Amsterdam: North Holland.

ZÜLCH, K. J. (1965) *Brain Tumors: Their Biology and Pathology,* 2nd American ed., trans. A. B. Rothballer and J. Olszewski. London: Heinemann.

ZÜLCH, K. J. (1971) *Atlas of the Histology of Brain Tumors.* Berlin: Springer Verlag (Text in six languages).

ZÜLCH, K. J. and WOOLF, A. L. (1964) Classification of brain tumors. *Acta neurochir.,* Suppl. X (Several authorities contribute papers).

The study and classification of tumours involving the central nervous system

The study of cerebral and spinal tumours based on a combination of naked-eye and microscopical examination can reasonably be said to have started with Virchow. Many of his observations are still as relevant and important today as when they were made; he observed, for instance, the lack of clear distinction between normal brain tissue and the edge of a glioma, and microscopically he could recognize the proliferation of both glial cells and glial fibres and the overgrowth of blood vessels.

During the second half of the nineteenth century there were rapid strides in histological technique and descriptions of different cerebral tumours were many. One of the first attempts to link the course of the disease observed clinically, with the morphology of the underlying growth, was that of Tooth (1912) who examined the neoplasms collected at The National Hospital, Queen Square, between the years 1902 and 1911. He conceived an ascending scale of malignancy up to sarcoma and stressed the prognostic importance of necrosis and vascular hyperplasia. The variety of appearances that gliomas present on microscopical examination he described as 'bewildering'.

A deliberate attempt to introduce order into the existing chaos was made by Bailey and Cushing (1926). They used the 'histogenetic' method of classifying glial tumours by their resemblance to embryological counterparts in normal development and proposed a scheme consisting of 14 main groups starting with medulloepithelioma as the most primitive and reaching the mature astrocytoma via the spongioblastoma (glioblastoma) and astroblastoma. Most subsequent attempts at classification have aimed at simplifying this scheme and deleting rarities (see Russell and Rubinstein (1971), Chapter 6). Del Rio-Hortega, however, used the metallic impregnation methods with which his name will always be associated, to classify tumours on the basis of details of their cell structure and processes and in 1933 presented an illustrated report. More recent accounts of gliomas examined with modifications of Hortega's techniques have been published by Polak (1966) and by Scharenberg and Liss (1969).

A different approach was adopted by Scherer, who between 1935 and 1940 published studies of brain tumours using whole brain slices processed in celloidin. He introduced the terms 'primary', 'secondary' and 'tertiary' structures. The primary structures of a glioma are the intrinsic formations characteristic of the tumour type, e.g. the rosettes of a medulloblastoma. Secondary structures comprise the increased concentrations of cells beyond the main body of the tumour, close to its advancing edges, particularly in subpial, subependymal or perivascular situations. Scherer emphasized the extent to which the architecture of gliomas was influenced by the existing structure of the nervous tissue and the way the shape of the tumour cells was determined by their surroundings. The tertiary structures include the excessive vascular proliferation and connective tissue scarring typical of a necrotic malignant glioma. Scherer did not, on the whole, applaud the classification of gliomas based solely on the appearances of individual cells and stressed the need for a 'complete' examination.

An attempt to simplify the diagnosis of gliomas by the use of a grading scheme (from I to IV) was advocated by Kernohan and Sayre (1952), who applied this system to astrocytomas (*see* p. 8), oligodendrogliomas and ependymomas. 'Glioblastoma multiforme' was replaced by 'astrocytoma grade IV' and certain of Bailey and Cushing's terms such as 'neuroepithelioma' were regarded as obsolete. The criteria used to place a tumour in a grade were principally the proportion of mature to immature cells, together with the frequency of mitotic figures, the degree of vascular changes and the presence of necrosis. But in practice it was found that 'grading' could not be applied to gliomas with the same facility and degree of accuracy that obtains, say, with carcinomas of the intestinal tract. Many authorities insist that 'grading' cannot be applied to small tumour biopsies at all, since the specimen obtained may not be representative of the whole of the growth, and argue that in any event purely cytological considerations are of no great value. A tumour labelled 'astrocytoma grade I' derived from the cerebral hemispheres of an adult is unlikely to behave in the same way as a cerebellar 'astrocytoma grade I' removed from a young person. The site of the growth and the age of the patient may be of more prognostic importance than the histological grade.

The term 'glioblastoma multiforme', though often synonymous with 'astrocytoma grade IV', remains in popular use. While it is clear that a good proportion of these tumours are anaplastic astrocytomas, others may be derived from oligodendrogliomas undergoing malignant changes and in some cases—the 'primary' glioblastomas—the entire tumour is formed by the proliferation of primitive glial cells with no indication of evolution from an earlier, more differentiated glioma. The features on which the diagnosis of glioblastoma depends are cellular pleomorphism with many primitive cells and a high incidence of mitotic division, necrosis of tumour tissue and extensive overgrowth of small blood vessels, usually with marked endothelial hyperplasia. A rare complication is for the increasingly florid vascular changes to become truly neoplastic and for a sarcoma of vascular mesodermal tissue to develop within the glioma. This composite glioblastoma–sarcoma is therefore of mixed neuroectodermal–mesodermal origin and presents a classification problem: in this Atlas we have placed it next to glioblastoma, regarding the sarcomatous element as a secondary effect.

The existence of such tumours of mixed type provides some of the more difficult problems of pathological diagnosis. Rubinstein (1972) distinguished three special forms of cell-mixture: the *mixed gliomas* containing more than one glial cell-type; the *gangliogliomas* in which neuronal and glial cells both participate; and the *glioma–sarcoma* which we have considered already. The first of these, the true mixed glioma, is exemplified by certain oligodendrogliomas containing varying numbers of astrocytes, often of primitive type, and such growths may be very difficult to distinguish from some 'pleomorphic' oligodendrogliomas, whose cells, despite their varied morphology, are all of oligodendrocytic origin. The second, ganglioglioma, must be diagnosed with some caution and only when careful pathological study has demonstrated that the neuronal elements in the growth are truly neoplastic. It is quite usual for an infiltrative astrocytoma to engulf any pre-existing neurons in its path and for them to remain embedded in the tumour substance without being destroyed.

Difficulties also commonly arise when gliomas invade the leptomeninges and stimulate a brisk growth of connective tissue in and around the cells sometimes with considerable morphological alteration. This form of growth is well known in medulloblastoma, where the bulk of the tumour may lie in the meninges and contain abundant reticulin fibrils, so much so that a diagnosis of arachnoidal sarcoma may be entertained. The controversy surrounding this interpretation is discussed in the appropriate section.

In the classification of lymphoreticular neoplasms (microglioma, reticulum cell sarcoma etc.) the present lack of clarity is reflected by the number of synonyms employed to describe what, in essence, is a proliferation of perivascular and meningeal primitive cells and of more mature microglia. We distinguish these primary tumours from the different type of involvement recognized in the systemic lymphomas.

Methods available for the study of tumours have increased in complexity in recent years. Cell and tissue culture techniques have been applied to CNS tumours for over forty years and much information obtained concerning the behaviour of cells *in vitro* (Lumsden 1971). Transplantation experiments using the brain or anterior chamber of the eye of animals have provided fresh insight into the *in vivo* growth of gliomas and into the phenomena of rejection. Electron-microscopical studies have been reported on almost all of the tumours portrayed in this Atlas and references to ultrastructural appearances have been included in the bibliographies. The study of enzyme histochemistry has revealed much detail of the metabolic activities of the tumours. Experimental induction of gliomas and nerve sheath tumours in animals has recently been facilitated by the advent of the potent *N*-nitroso compounds. However, details of these developing fields of research lie outside the scope of this Atlas.

Bibliography

BAILEY, P. and CUSHING, H. (1926) See p. x.

KERNOHAN, J. W. and SAYRE, G. P. (1952) *Tumors of the Central Nervous System. Atlas of Tumor Pathology.* Fascicle 35. Washington, D.C.: Armed Forces Institute of Pathology.

LUMSDEN, C. E. (1971) The study by tissue culture of tumours of the CNS. In *Pathology of Tumours of the Nervous System*, ed. Dorothy S. Russell and L. J. Rubinstein, 3rd ed., pp. 334–420. London: Edward Arnold.

POLAK, M. (1966) *Blastomas del Sistema Nervioso Central y Periferico.* Buenos Aires: Lopez.

DEL RIO-HORTEGA, P. (1933) *The Microscopic Anatomy of Tumors of the Central and Peripheral Nervous System*, trans. A. Pineda, G. V. Russell and K. M. Earle (1962). Springfield, Ill.: Charles C Thomas.

RUSSELL, DOROTHY S. and RUBINSTEIN, L. J. (1971) See p. x.

RUBINSTEIN, L. J. (1972) See p. x.

SCHARENBERG, K. and LISS, L. (1969) *Neuroectodermal Tumors of the Central and Peripheral Nervous System.* Baltimore: Williams and Wilkins.

SCHERER, H. J. (1940) *Brain*, **63**, 1 (Summarizes previous work).

TOOTH, H. H. (1912) *Brain*, **35**, 71.

The cells of the central nervous system: their normal and pathological appearances

The cells of the central nervous system comprise the neurons, neuroglia (astrocytes, oligodendrocytes and ependyma) and microglia. The brain and spinal cord are composed of an elaborate network of these cell bodies and cell processes, covered by the delicate pia mater and arachnoid (leptomeninges), and protected externally by the fibrous dura mater (pachymeninx).

Neurons vary considerably in shape and size; for example, the granule cells of the cerebellum are less than a tenth of the size of their neighbours, the Purkinje cells. But certain essential features are common to all. The cell body has one single afferent process —the axon—and a variable, often large, number of efferents—the dendrites. Each neuron is an individual and irreplaceable part of the whole nervous system, its 'uniqueness' depending upon its synaptic connections. Large neurons have large nuclei, containing prominent single nucleoli, and the cytoplasm contains the characteristic blocks of basophilic material known as 'Nissl substance'. Smaller neurons (with shorter axons) have much less Nissl substance.

The neuroglial (= nerve glue) cells were originally considered to be the connective tissue ('glueing together tissue') of the brain.

The astrocytes (star-shaped cells) are subdivided into protoplasmic (found in grey matter) and fibrillary (grey and white matter) types. With Cajal's gold sublimate preparation both types are seen to have a sucker foot attached to a capillary, but the fibrillary astrocytes contain intracytoplasmic neuroglial fibrils and their processes are longer, finer and more numerous than those of the protoplasmic. The astrocytes of the granular layer of the cerebellum are known as Bergmann cells.

The nucleus of the normal astrocyte, as seen in haematoxylin–eosin preparations, is oval and vesicular, smaller than that of a neuron and without a nucleolus. The cytoplasm is usually indistinct and small in amount.

Under pathological conditions—infection, anoxia, infarction, tumour-formation— astrocytes can react with 'progressive' or 'regressive' changes. In the former the cell-body swells, the nucleus enlarges and may be placed towards one end of a clearly defined mass of eosinophil cytoplasm. The term 'gemistocytic' (derived from the Greek verb meaning to fill or load) is in common use to describe these swollen astrocytes (Plate 1, Fig. 2). In very unfavourable conditions degenerative or 'regressive' changes are found: the astrocytic processes break off ('clasmatodendrosis'); the cell-body becomes granular and the nucleus pyknotic.

Oligodendrocytes are normally very numerous in the white matter and are found in the grey as perineuronal satellites. They have small, regular, round nuclei (Plate 1, Fig. 3).

Plate 1. THE CELLS OF THE CNS

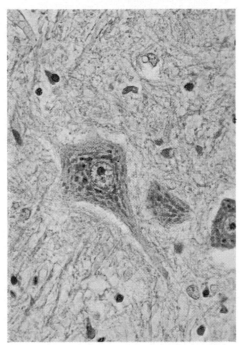

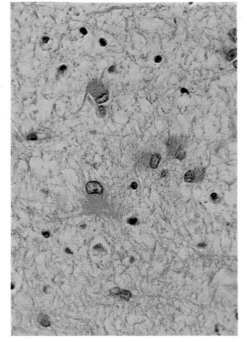

Fig. 1. A large neuron from the oculomotor nucleus. The nucleus contains a darkly stained nucleolus. Large blocks of basophil material (Nissl granules) are present in the cytoplasm. Portions of two other neurons are also seen. (H & E × 420)

Fig. 2. Gemistocytic astrocytes. These cells have large vesicular nuclei and masses of eosinophil cytoplasm. Fibre formation is evident. The small, dark nuclei are oligodendrocytes. (H & E × 420)

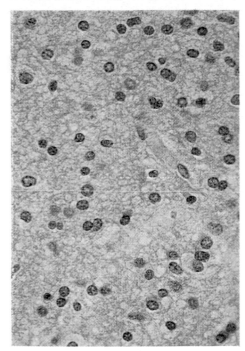

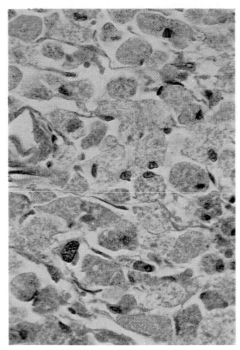

Fig. 3. Oligodendrocytes. The cells have round nuclei of regular size and sometimes are paired. A small clear perinuclear zone indicates 'acute swelling'. (H & E × 420)

Fig. 4. Cerebral histiocytes (microglia) engaged in active phagocytosis, with granular material inside their distended cytoplasm. Several dark, elongated rod cells (hypertrophic microglia) are also present. (H & E × 420)

Like the Schwann cells of the peripheral nervous system, their prime concern is the formation and maintenance of the myelin sheath that covers the axon. As their name implies, they have few glial processes. In various degenerative conditions oligodendrocytes react with 'acute swelling'. The nuclei come to lie near the centre of the distended, but clear, cytoplasm and the processes disappear. The cell-membrane remains well-defined. These appearances are recapitulated in the oligodendrogliomas.

The ependymal cells which line the ventricular cavities, aqueduct and central canal of the spinal cord are ciliated and resemble columnar epithelium. They possess tiny rod-shaped 'blepharoplasts' (*see* p. 44) which at the electron-microscopical level have been identified as the basal bodies in which the ciliary shafts terminate.

The microglia do not share the common neuroectodermal origin of the neuroglia, being of mesodermal derivation. Their separation from the other elements of the nervous system was the work of del Rio-Hortega and in consequence they are sometimes known as 'Hortega cells'. They are the representatives of the reticuloendothelial system in the brain and can act as phagocytes (Plate 1, Fig. 4). Normally they have small, inconspicuous oval or bean-shaped nuclei and fine branching processes revealed only by metallic impregnations. Under some conditions, e.g. dementia paralytica, the microglia elongate and lose their branching processes (rod-cells). Where there is debris, phagocytosis takes place and the cells quickly adopt a rounded form as the cytoplasm is filled with the ingested material.

Neuroepithelial tumours:
a simplified scheme of classification

1. *Glial*

   (*a*) Astrocytoma

       i. differentiated:
   >protoplasmic
   >gemistocytic
   >fibrillary
   >piloid (pilocytic)
   >mixed

       ii. malignant (anaplastic), usually of mixed composition, shades into glioblastoma

   (*b*) Glioblastoma

   (*c*) Oligodendroglioma:
   >typical
   >atypical
   >malignant (polymorphous)

   (*d*) Ependymoma
   >myxopapillary ependymoma of filum terminale
   >ependymoblastoma
   >subependymoma

   (*e*) Choroid plexus papilloma

2. *Primitive bipotential*

   (*a*) Medulloblastoma

3. *Neuronal and neuroglial*

   (*a*) Gangliocytoma

   (*b*) Ganglioglioma

   (*c*) Neuroblastoma

ASTROCYTOMA

Tumours of astrocytic origin are relatively common. They may be highly differentiated and slowly growing, or rapidly destructive and anaplastic. They may be found in the cerebral hemispheres, brain-stem, cerebellum or spinal cord. In adults astrocytomas are usually diffuse tumours involving the cerebral hemispheres and are malignant judged by both cytological appearances and clinical behaviour. Russell and Rubinstein noted anaplasia in some 80 per cent of their specimens. The small temporal lobe tumours (Cavanagh 1958) are exceptional and closer in character to hamartomas. In children and adolescents benign astrocytomas of the piloid type may involve the cerebellum and the region of the third ventricle, and the common site for a malignant astrocytoma is the pons.

Astrocytomas are classified on microscopical appearances into (a) protoplasmic, (b) gemistocytic, (c) fibrillary, (d) piloid (pilocytic) and (e) malignant (anaplastic) types.

The uncommon protoplasmic astrocytoma is usually honeycombed with cysts, and the cells have small nuclei of regular size lying in a matrix containing relatively few glial fibres. The gemistocytic astrocytoma (see Plate 7, Figs 1, 2) is formed of globular cells with eccentric nuclei and abundant eosinophilic cytoplasm. It is seldom benign. The fibrillary astrocytoma is characterized by numerous coarse or fine fibrils, often of considerable length, well demonstrated by the use of the phosphotungstic acid–haematoxylin (PTAH) stain. The piloid (pilocytic) astrocytoma is made up of cells with narrow oval nuclei and elongated fibrillary processes tending to lie in parallel bundles. Often, loose-textured microcystic areas are found adjacent to dense fibrillary growth. Rosenthal fibres (thick eosinophil carrot-shaped fibrous structures) and granular bodies (intracytoplasmic droplets) are characteristic. These tumours are frequently calcified, and are the most slowly growing and benign form of astrocytoma. Included in this category are the cerebellar astrocytoma, the 'juvenile' type of astrocytoma of the third ventricle, and the optic nerve glioma. The term 'polar spongioblastoma' has been used for astrocytomas of this type by certain authors (e.g. Zülch 1965; Ringertz and Nordenstam 1951) and confusion may arise since this term also denotes a rare, malignant glioma of childhood (see p. 147). Anaplastic (malignant) astrocytomas showing hypercellularity, pleomorphism, increased mitotic activity and focal necrosis are common, and shade towards glioblastoma multiforme; endothelial hyperplasia of blood vessels is a constant feature.

In von Recklinghausen's neurofibromatosis the various types of astrocytic glioma that may be encountered include diffuse gliomatosis of the cerebrum or cerebellum (see Plate 4, Figs 2–4), optic nerve gliomas and pilocytic astrocytomas of the third ventricle. In tuberose sclerosis giant-celled subependymal astrocytomas are sometimes found, and these tumours tend to follow a benign course despite the striking appearance of the giant gemistocytic astrocytes that usually form the bulk of the cell population. It is likely that the growths arise in the subependymal nodules of abnormal glia typical of this disease.

Optic nerve gliomas may be solitary or be found as one of the various manifestations of neurofibromatosis. The most usual type of appearance is of slender fibrillated astrocytes in bundles within the substance of the nerve (see Plate 5, Figs 1–3) but in some examples oligodendroglial cells form an important component of a truly 'mixed' glioma.

It is in the tumours of the astrocyte series that the system of 'grading' can be applied with the best results. The scheme proposed by Kernohan et al. (1949) recognizes four classes in ascending order of malignancy. Grade I includes the most benign astrocytomas with the best prognosis (in practice mainly cerebellar). All the cells in these growths should resemble normal astrocytes; mitotic figures, blood vessel changes and necrosis are never found. In Grade II some pleomorphism of the cells is permitted, though almost all are typical astrocytes; minimal vascular changes only, and no necrosis should be present. The cellularity of the tumour is comparable with that of normal brain tissue. A much more varied appearance is characteristic of Grade III, with some 50 per cent of the cells 'anaplastic'. The tumour is hypercellular, with some mitotic figures; blood vessels are hyperplastic with prominent endothelia and some necrosis of the tissue is usually found. Grade IV astrocytoma (including glioblastoma multiforme) is typified by cellular anaplasia and pleomorphism, with numerous mitotic figures, marked vascular changes and necrosis of the tumour that may be extensive. The prognosis is poor.

The convenience of this system, relating microscopical appearance to prognosis, has led to its widespread popularity amongst clinicians and pathologists. Despite its inherent limitations—particularly the danger of regarding a small needle-biopsy specimen as typical of the whole of a large glioma—the grading scheme is likely to continue in use.

Bibliography

CAVANAGH, J. B. (1958) *Brain*, **81,** 389 (Small gliomas in temporal lobe).
DAVIS, R. L. (1971) In *Pathology of the Nervous System*, ed. J. Minckler, vol. 2, p. 2001. New York: McGraw-Hill.
ELVIDGE, A. R. (1968) *J. Neurosurg.*, **28,** 399 (Long-term follow-up and survival).
GRCEVIC, N. and YATES, P. O. (1957) *J. Path. Bact.*, **73,** 467 (Rosenthal fibres in CNS tumours).
HERNDON, R. M., RUBINSTEIN, L. J., FREEMAN, J. M. and MATHIESON, G. (1970) *J. Neuropath. exp. Neurol.*, **29,** 524 (Rosenthal fibres in Alexander's disease and multiple sclerosis; ultrastructure).
HOYT, W. F., MESHEL, L. G., LESSELL, S., SCHATZ, N. J. and SUCKLING, R. D. (1973) *Brain*, **96,** 121 (Malignant optic glioma).
KERNOHAN, J. W., MABON, R. F., SVIEN, H. J. and ADSON, W. A. (1949) *Proc. Staff Meet. Mayo Clin.*, **24,** 71.
LEVY, L. F. and ELVIDGE, A. R. (1956) *J. Neurosurg.*, **13,** 413 (Review of 176 cases).
NEVIN, S. (1938) *Brain*, **61,** 170 (Diffuse gliomatosis).
RINGERTZ, N. and NORDENSTAM, H. (1951) *J. Neuropath. exp. Neurol.*, **10,** 343 (Cerebellar astrocytoma).
RUSSELL, DOROTHY S. and RUBINSTEIN, L. J. (1971) See p. x.
SCHERER, H. J. (1940) *Am. J. Cancer*, **40,** 159 (A study of cerebral astrocytomas, emphasizing their diffuseness).
ZÜLCH, K. J. (1965) See p. x.

ASTROCYTOMA

Case 1. Woman aged 45

History. Six months' headache, bifrontal spreading to left parietal and occipital areas; often worse on waking in the morning; for three months, vomiting in the evening every three to four days. Some impairment of recent memory and difficulty in expressing herself.

Examination. Dysphasia, particularly on nomination; dyscalculia; dyspraxia. Chronic papilloedema without haemorrhages or exudates. Mild upper motor neuron paresis of the right side of the face and proximally in the arm.

Investigations. Scintiscan revealed area of uptake 4 cm in diameter subcortically in left frontal lobe. Carotid angiogram: large posterior frontal tumour, avascular and probably cystic. External carotid injection showed no filling from the dura mater.

Clinical diagnosis. Cystic glioma most likely; meningioma probably excluded by contrast studies.

Operation. Left frontal craniotomy revealed swollen yellowish cortex in the middle frontal convolution. Aspirating needle encountered irregular resistance throughout the frontal lobe, with two cysts: one containing 10 ml yellow fluid and the second 2 ml. Frontal lobectomy was performed back to the level of the genu of the corpus callosum, but it was clear that the tumour infiltrated behind the level of the excision.

Follow-up. Postoperatively the patient did well, with clearing of the dysphasia, but her symptoms returned within two months and she died one month later.

Necropsy. The entire frontal lobectomy site was filled with recurrent neoplasm.

Microscopical appearances

The tumour is composed of a delicate cobweb-like matrix of fine and coarse neuroglial fibrils in which small oval nuclei are diffusely disposed. Some cells resemble gemistocytic astrocytes, with swollen cytoplasm. There are no mitoses. Blood vessels are mostly small and thin-walled. Scattered within the tumour substance are some normal neurons.

Diagnosis. Protoplasmic and fibrillary astrocytoma.

Summary

The appearances of this well-differentiated astrocytoma (corresponding to Grade II) suggested a slow tempo of growth. The rapidity of the recurrence, and its extent, were unexpected, although it was obvious that the excision was incomplete. Astrocytomas in the cerebral hemispheres of adults are seldom truly benign; they are prone to focal anaplasia and their rate of growth is variable: in some cases recurrence is rapid.

Plate 2. ASTROCYTOMA

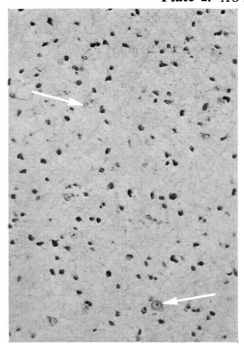

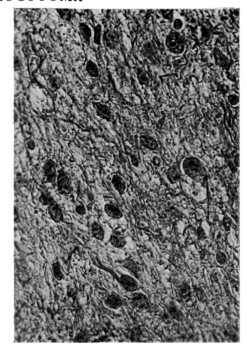

Fig. 1 (Case 1). In this field there are only moderate numbers of tumour cells; their nuclei are small, oval or triangular, and of fairly regular size. They lie in a finely reticulated network in which several neurons are recognized (arrows). (H & E × 210)

Fig. 2 (Case 1). Glial fibrils are numerous, and form a dense network between the nuclei. (PTAH × 530)

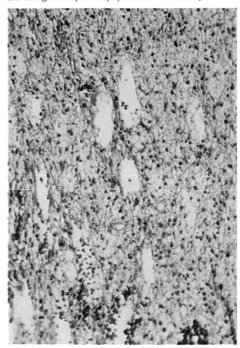

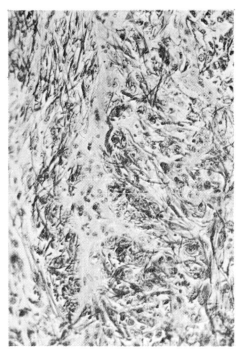

Fig. 3 (Case 1). There are multiple small cysts amongst the tumour cells, many of which possess fine, or coarser, fibrillary processes. (PTAH × 130)

Fig. 4. In this astrocytoma the perivascular cells have numerous, abnormally thick glial fibres. (PTAH × 210)

ASTROCYTOMA

Case 2. Schoolgirl aged 13, with an excellent past school record

History. Six months' tiredness. Five months' occipital headaches, associated with vomiting at first succeeding, but later preceding, the onset of the headache which was manifest as a severe pain in the occiput and back of the neck particularly marked at night. Lost 16 kg (35 lb) in weight. One month's unsteady gait, needed support when walking. Sudden turning of head precipitated giddiness. Attacks of diplopia lasting a few minutes occurred frequently.

Examination. Thin and ill, but with normal intellect. Pain in neck on full rotation to either direction. Mild papilloedema in both fundi without haemorrhages or exudates. Grade III nystagmus to left; grade I to right; also vertical nystagmus. Hypotonia of all four limbs, particularly on left. Cerebellar incoordination left arm and leg with impairment of rapid repetitive movements in these limbs. Gait ataxic, veering to the left; unable to walk heel to toe.

Investigations. Skull radiograph revealed erosion of anterior and posterior clinoids and dorsum sellae. Sutures wider than normal. Ventriculogram disclosed symmetrical hydrocephalus with kinking and displacement of the aqueduct and fourth ventricle to the right by a large left cerebellar mass.

Clinical diagnosis lay between medulloblastoma and cystic astrocytoma. The length of history, with the presence of a mass laterally in the hemisphere rather than in the vermis, favoured the latter.

Operation. Left unilateral cerebellar craniotomy revealed a cyst containing 20 ml of clear yellow fluid. Incision showed a solid purple-grey mass of tissue extending from the cyst wall to the superior and lateral aspects of the hemisphere measuring 3·5 cm in diameter. It was completely excised with a surrounding fringe of white matter.

Follow-up. She made an excellent recovery. No radiotherapy was given. Seven years later she remains well without neurological signs.

Microscopical appearances

The tumour tissue is in part loose-textured, containing multiple cysts, while in part it is compact. In the compact regions the pattern of the growth is of interlacing bundles of elongated fibrillated cells and Rosenthal fibres are numerous. Many of the smaller blood vessels are ensheathed by bundles of fibrillated astrocytes, mainly lying in a longitudinal axis. In the nearby cerebellum there is dense isomorphic gliosis.

Diagnosis. Cerebellar astrocytoma of piloid (pilocytic) type.

Summary

The piloid cerebellar astrocytoma, particularly common in childhood and adolescence, has a very much better prognosis than any other astrocytic tumour and the distinction from the highly malignant medulloblastoma, which in some cases can only be made with certainty by microscopical study, is vital. Sometimes it may be difficult to distinguish a cystic cerebellar astrocytoma, containing altered blood, from a gliotic haemangioblastoma cerebelli (*see* p. 78), particularly if only small pieces of the latter, lacking the typical architecture, are submitted for study.

Plate 3. ASTROCYTOMA

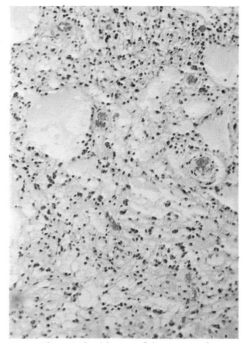

Fig. 1 (Case 2). In this part of the tumour there are numerous small cysts containing pink-staining liquid and some thin-walled vessels congested with blood. The astrocytic nuclei vary slightly in size and shape. (H & E   × 105)

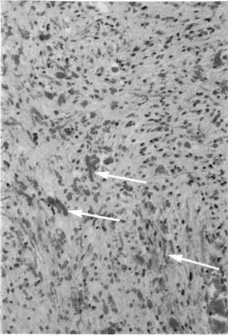

Fig. 2 (Case 2). Rosenthal fibres (arrows) are of varied configuration and tend to stain bright red with eosin. (H & E   × 130)

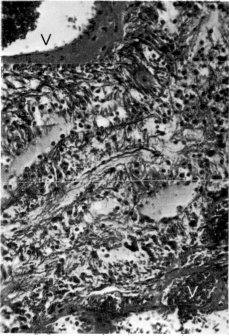

Fig. 3 (Case 2). The nuclei are regular, but glial fibres vary in length and thickness. There are several small cysts. Blood vessels (v) are thickened. (PTAH   × 105)

ASTROCYTOMA
Case 3. Woman aged 58

History. Six months' progressive mental deterioration, headaches and unsteady gait.

Examination. Unable to understand more than simple commands. Slight nominal dysphasia. Impairment of voluntary gaze in all directions with bilateral ptosis. Spastic tetraparesis. Blood pressure 150/90. Numerous pedunculated nodules and *café-au-lait* spots in the skin (one of her three children was also noted to have skin nodules).

Investigations. Carotid angiogram indicated ventricular dilatation. Myodil ventriculogram confirmed the symmetrical hydrocephalus and showed the aqueduct to be narrow and irregular, possibly as a result of infiltrative tumour.

Clinical diagnosis. An intrinsic tumour of the brain-stem appeared likely, but exploration to exclude an anterior extracerebral mass such as an acoustic nerve tumour was undertaken.

Operation. Right posterior temporoparietal craniotomy and transtentorial exposure of front of brain-stem. No extracerebral tumour was found. The patient died one day later.

Necropsy. Multiple neurofibromatosis; diffuse glioma of thalamus; glioma of mid-brain; gliomatous nodules of cerebellum; bilateral phaeochromocytoma of adrenal.

Microscopical appearances

In the thalamus and in the mid-brain there is diffuse infiltration by astrocytoma composed of cells with slender oval nuclei and fibrils of varied length. Around the aqueduct the tumour is densely packed with glial fibres abundant. In the cerebellum the nodules are piloid astrocytoma with bundles of fine fibrils streaming through the molecular layer onto the pial surface.

Diagnosis. Multiple astrocytomas; phaeochromocytoma; von Recklinghausen's neurofibromatosis.

Summary

Clinical opinion in this case strongly favoured an intrinsic brain-stem tumour, but the possibility of an extracerebral mass had to be considered.

The manifestations of multiple neurofibromatosis are many, and can occur in any combination. It is often stated that in cases where the peripheral lesions are numerous the central ones are sparse, but this does not always hold good. Glial tumours are usually astrocytomas of pilocytic type, but ependymomas and meningiomas may be found as well as the neurofibromas of cranial and spinal roots.

Phaeochromocytoma of the adrenal is a well-recognized feature of multiple neurofibromatosis. The growths may be unilateral or bilateral and may be physiologically inactive or responsible for systemic hypertension from the secretion of pressor amines.

Plate 4. ASTROCYTOMA

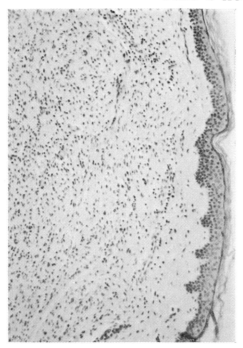

Fig. 1 (Case 3). Skin: neurofibroma. The epidermis covers a cellular mass composed of elongated cells with oval nuclei lying in a fibrous matrix. (H & E × 105)

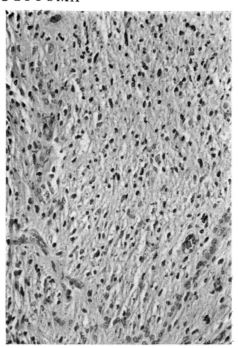

Fig. 2 (Case 3). Thalamic tumour: fibrillary astrocytes with long, thin or plump oval nuclei. Blood vessels are inconspicuous. (H & E × 130)

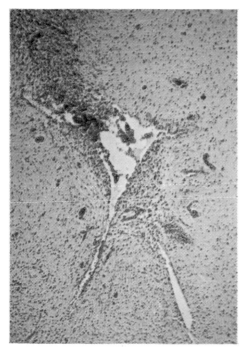

Fig. 3 (Case 3). The aqueduct is deformed by gliomatous infiltration of the surrounding subependymal tissues, and the tumour shades away diffusely into the surroundings. (PTAH × 45)

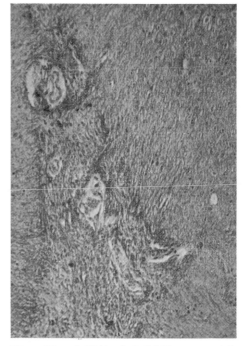

Fig. 4 (Case 3). 'Bridges' of glial fibres connect the cerebellum with the densely infiltrated leptomeninges. (PTAH × 105)

OPTIC GLIOMA
Case 4. Girl aged 6

History. Two months' bilateral frontal headaches associated with nausea. Her gait, at the same time, became increasingly unsteady. Mother noticed that her pupils had enlarged by approximately one and a half times.

Examination. Drowsy, disorientated. Five *café-au-lait* marks within a 5 cm area of skin. No papilloedema. Both pupils dilated. Bilateral extensor plantar responses.

Investigations. Skull radiograph suggested chronic raised intracranial pressure. Right carotid angiogram indicated marked symmetrical hydrocephalus. Ventriculograms revealed great thickening of the optic nerves and chiasm. Air encephalograms showed an irregular mass encroaching upon the anterior aspect of the third ventricle.

Operation. Left frontal craniotomy. Both optic nerves and chiasm were greatly thickened (optic nerve 12 mm diameter) and vascular. A small biopsy was taken from the right nerve.

Follow-up. Ventriculocaval shunt was required to drain both lateral ventricles, following which the patient became normally alert. She was given radiotherapy. One year later she was well and making good progress at school.

Microscopical appearances

The morsel of tissue removed is made up of small cells with small oval nuclei lying in an eosinophil matrix. Only with PTAH staining is the intense fibrillary network visible. Elongated fine hair-like fibres course in close-packed bundles (piloid type).

Diagnosis. Optic nerve glioma (piloid astrocytoma).

Summary

In this patient the presence of *café-au-lait* spots strongly suggests that the optic glioma is part of a *'forme fruste'* of neurofibromatosis. It may well be that no other lesions will ever be manifest. Many optic gliomas are thought to arise on a hamartomatous basis; it may be that some examples are not truly neoplastic lesions.

The cellular composition of the optic glioma has long been controversial: some authorities regard the tumour as oligodendroglial, others as astrocytic. Some tumours, certainly, are mixed. Our Case 4 is a typical example and the growth is predominantly of elongated fibrillary astrocytes.

Plate 5. ASTROCYTOMA

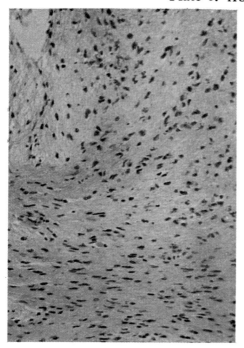

Fig. 1 (Case 4). Small oval and elongated astrocytic nuclei in an eosinophil matrix. (H & E × 210)

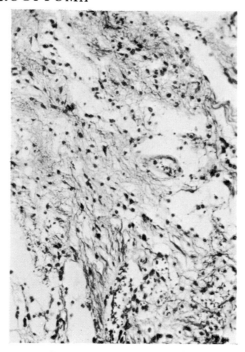

Fig. 2 (Case 4). Numerous fine hair-like processes in this piloid astrocytoma. (PTAH × 210)

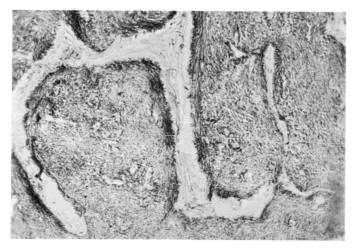

Fig. 3. A *post mortem* specimen of an optic glioma. The bundles of nerve fibres are swollen from diffuse infiltration and present an exaggerated appearance. The patient had neurofibromatosis. (PTAH × 105)

ASTROCYTOMA

Case 5. Girl aged 5: normal birth and development

History. Four months' unsteady gait, worsening progressively. Two months' speaking and swallowing became slow. One month's tremor of both hands.

Examination. Bilateral fifth, left third and left seventh lower motor neuron nerve palsies. Lateral nystagmus. Slurred speech. Ataxia of all limbs and bilateral pyramidal deficit with left extensor plantar response; gait ataxic. Romberg's sign present (falling to right).

Investigations. Left vertebral angiogram indicated a mass in the brain-stem spreading into the left middle cerebellar peduncle with no abnormal circulation. Air ventriculogram showed symmetrical hydrocephalus with displacement backward of the fourth ventricle and deformation and splaying of its floor by an encroaching mass in the brain-stem.

Clinical diagnosis. Pontine glioma.

Operation. Exploration of the posterior fossa confirmed that the floor of the fourth ventricle was grossly widened, and 'humped' on left side but no tumour lay in the floor. No biopsy was obtained.

Follow-up. Following a course of radiotherapy the child's condition was greatly improved. She became almost normal apart from bilateral sixth nerve palsy. Three months later she deteriorated with headache, vomiting and disordered eye movements and bilateral fifth and seventh nerve palsies. After a further two months she died. The total duration of illness was eleven months.

Necropsy. The pons was greatly enlarged (6·5 cm across); on section fibre-bundles were separated by ill-defined masses of firm grey tissue.

Microscopical appearances

The tumour is diffusely infiltrative, tending to run between the pontine fibre-bundles, pushing them apart. The cell-type is varied: there are elongated spindle-cells, small astrocytes and closely packed masses of primitive cells with dark-staining oval nuclei, sometimes ranged about necrotic zones in 'pseudo-palisade' formation. Mitotic figures are present. In places the tissue is semicystic.

Diagnosis. Diffuse malignant astrocytoma of pons.

Summary

The pons is a common site for a malignant astrocytoma in childhood, but is rarely affected in adults. The growth is usually diffuse, producing enlargement ('hypertrophy') without obliteration of the fibre-bundles. The prognosis is always poor, but the course of the illness may be protracted and extended over several years.

Plate 6. ASTROCYTOMA

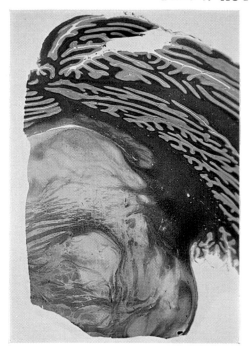

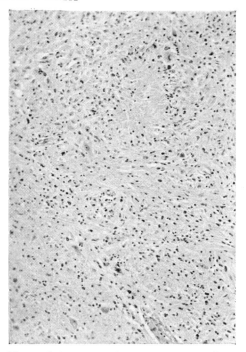

Fig. 1 (Case 5). The section includes one cerebellar hemisphere and one half of the pons. The pons is greatly enlarged. The cerebellum is compressed and the fourth ventricle reduced to a slit. With this method of staining the pontine fibre-bundles appear blue-black; between and around them the neoplastic tissue is pale. (Heidenhain's myelin   × 2)

Fig. 2. Infiltrative malignant astrocytoma. Some remaining pontine neurons can be recognized. (H & E   × 105)

ASTROCYTOMA
Case 6. Woman aged 58

History. Six weeks' rapidly progressive mental deterioration with failure of memory, loss of interest and insight. No headache or vomiting.

Examination. Alert, but demented, uncooperative and confused with fluctuating jargon dysphasia; papilloedema more marked on the right than the left; right facio-brachial weakness.

Investigations. Electroencephalogram indicated a left temporal focus. Left carotid angiogram showed a posterior frontal lesion and its position, low in the frontal lobe, was defined by air ventriculogram.

Clinical diagnosis. Glioma more likely than metastasis or abscess.

Operation. Left frontal craniotomy. The frontal lobe was bulging and much of its inferior surface replaced by pink, friable tumour. It was clear that it infiltrated widely; enough was removed to lower the intracranial tension.

Follow-up. The patient died three days later.

Microscopical appearances

The biopsy is of a tumour many of whose cells are globoid in shape. They possess eccentric, oval, vesicular nuclei and large masses of eosinophil cytoplasm. With PTAH-staining fine neuroglial fibres are plentiful. In one region purulent necrosis, endothelial hyperplasia of blood vessels, cellular pleomorphism and mitotic figures indicate malignant change.

Diagnosis. Malignant gemistocytic astrocytoma (corresponding to Grade III).

Summary

The rapid progression of mental symptoms with angiographic evidence of space-occupation pointed to a malignant tumour. There was nothing to suggest a metastasis: it proved to be a glioma extending widely through the frontal lobe.

Malignant astrocytomas are common in the cerebral hemispheres and usually are composed of cells of varied appearance: the 'pure' gemistocytic astrocytoma is not frequently encountered. Despite the general uniformity of cell-type, focal anaplasia and necrosis establish the malignancy of this tumour.

Plate 7. ASTROCYTOMA

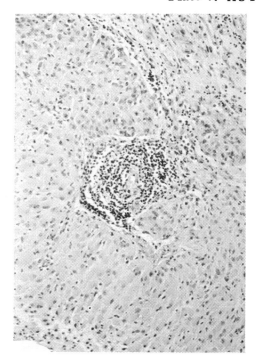

Fig. 1 (Case 6). The tumour is composed of a closely packed mass of cells with distinct, eosinophil cytoplasm and eccentrically placed nuclei. There are foci of perivascular lymphocytic cuffing. (H & E × 210)

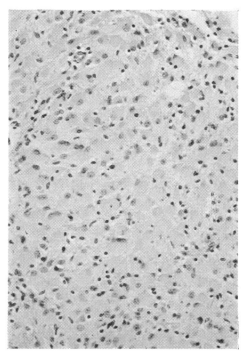

Fig. 2 (Case 6). The tumour cells are typical gemistocytic astrocytes with oval nuclei and plentiful eosinophil cytoplasm. (H & E × 210)

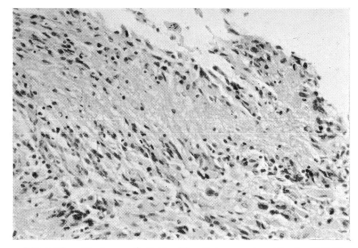

Fig. 3 (Case 6). A necrotic zone with cellular pseudo-pallisade. (H & E × 210)

ASTROCYTOMA

Case 7. Man aged 22

History. Five years' fits. At first momentary episodes of 'unawareness' occurring once a day; then for three years additional attacks with loss of consciousness and jerking of all limbs which were controlled with phenobarbitone. For two years headaches, lasting up to two hours. Five months' progressive weakness of left arm and leg.

Examination. Bilateral severe chronic papilloedema. Left spastic hemiparesis, predominantly in arm with left extensor plantar response.

Investigations. Skull radiograph showed evidence of raised pressure. Scintiscan demonstrated increased uptake in the right upper parietal zone extending up to the midline. Carotid angiogram (bilateral) indicated a large, deep, frontoparietal mass with neoplastic circulation with arteriovenous communications.

Clinical diagnosis. Malignant glioma.

Operation. Right posterior frontal craniotomy. No cyst was found, but an infiltrative tumour, partly soft, partly hard and very vascular, presented on the surface, extending across the posterior frontal lobe to the falx medially. A palliative subtotal removal was obtained.

Follow-up. Following surgery and a course of radiotherapy the patient's headache and left-sided weakness improved. One year later he deteriorated again and died.

Microscopical appearances

The appearances of the tumour vary from that of a microcystic astrocytoma to that of a highly malignant glioma with cellular pleomorphism, abnormal mitotic figures, zones of necrosis and vascular hyperplasia. The transition is clear-cut. In the first type of tissue the cells are small gemistocytic astrocytes associated with fine fibrils; in the second there are monstrous giant cells with large single nuclei or multiple nuclei, elongated perivascular primitive cells and, indeed, cells of every variety of shape and size.

Diagnosis. Astrocytoma with transition to glioblastoma (giant-cell type).

Summary

The evolution of malignant astrocytoma and glioblastoma multiforme from existing cerebral astrocytomas is well recognized. Russell and Rubinstein (1971, p. 126) found that in 75 per cent of a series of ninety-eight astrocytomas malignant changes were evident, and that in nearly a half of these cases (thirty-four) the diagnosis was frank glioblastoma.

In this case the five year's history of fits, with the recent onset of hemiparesis, is in accord with the pathological finding of a malignant tumour supervening upon a more benign one.

Plate 8. ASTROCYTOMA

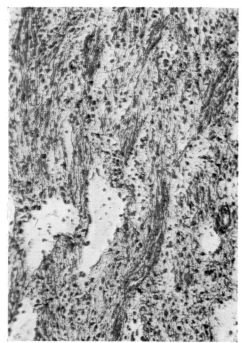

Fig. 1 (Case 7). Astrocytoma of 'benign' appearance, with small cysts and finely fibrillated cells. (PTAH × 130)

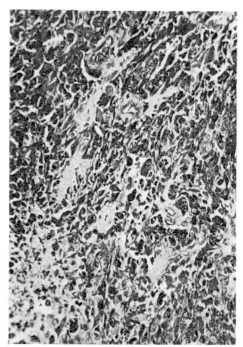

Fig. 2 (Case 7). Malignant astrocytoma with hyper-cellularity, pleomorphism and prominent small blood vessels. (PTAH × 175)

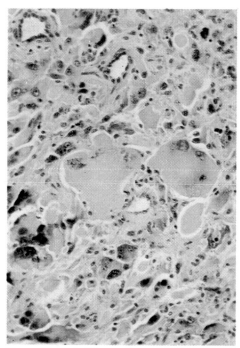

Fig. 3 (Case 7). Bizarre giant cells with multiple nuclei. (H van Gieson × 175)

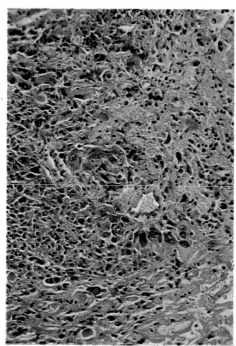

Fig. 4 (Case 7). Some of the monster cells have prominent nucleoli and, to some extent, resemble neurons. (H van Gieson × 105)

GLIOBLASTOMA MULTIFORME

This is considered the most malignant of the gliomas involving adults and corresponds to 'astrocytoma Grade IV' of Kernohan's grading. The tumours are often large and partly necrotic, infiltrating and destroying considerable amounts of white matter in the hemispheres (Plate 9, Fig. 1) and may involve both sides of the brain, spreading via the corpus callosum ('butterfly glioma'). They are less common in the posterior part of the cerebrum than the anterior, and relatively rare in the cerebellum, brain-stem and spinal cord. To the naked eye they present a varied pattern of grey solid tumour tissue, in places speckled red with haemorrhage, alternating with portions that are soft, yellow and necrotic.

Microscopically they are characterized by cellular pleomorphism, vascular endothelial hyperplasia and the presence of zones of necrosis bordered by small primitive glial cells in 'pseudo-palisades' (see Plates 10 and 11). Perhaps the most typical cells are slender, elongated primitive cells with fine processes extending from each pole, but more memorable are the 'monstrous' giant cells with very large single or multiple nuclei, though these are not an invariable feature. While in some cases many microscopical fields have such a varied cellular content that the term 'multiforme' is extremely appropriate, other cases of more uniform appearance, some entirely 'microcellular', nonetheless carry the same poor prognosis. In some glioblastomas mitotic figures are frequent and abnormal 'granular' forms may be found (Swaen et al. 1964). When the giant cells predominate the tumour may be referred to as a 'giant cell glioblastoma'. These are usually circumscribed and, in the experience of some authors, may be associated with a better than average prognosis if adequately treated. This subtype includes the growths interpreted as 'monstrocellular sarcoma'.

It has been accepted that glioblastomas may arise as the result of anaplasia in pre-existing astrocytomas (and oligodendrogliomas), or may appear spontaneously with nothing to suggest a pre-existing differentiated glioma.

One feature that is striking is the excessive formation of new blood vessels often extending beyond the confines of the tumour (see Plate 11, Fig. 2). These are often in the form of disorderly tangles or 'glomeruloid' masses of capillaries with large, prominent endothelial cells, among which mitotic figures may be found. This vascular hyperplasia may be of any degree up to malignant neoplasia when the resulting mixed tumour can properly be termed 'glioblastoma-sarcoma' (see Plate 12, Figs 1–4).

Bibliography

BATZDORF, U. and MALAMUD, N. (1963) *J. Neurosurg.*, **20**, 122 (Multifocal glioblastoma: incidence).
EADE, O. E. and URICH, H. (1971) *J. Path.*, **103**, 245 (CSF spread).
FEIGIN, I., ALLEN, L. B., LIPKIN, L. and GROSS, J. W. (1958) *Cancer*, **11**, 264 (Sarcomatous transformation of vascular endothelium).
MANUELIDIS, E. E. and SOLITARE, G. B. (1971) In *Pathology of the Nervous System*, ed. J. Minckler, vol. 2, 2026. New York: McGraw-Hill.
NYSTRÖM, S. (1960) *Acta path. microbiol. scand.*, **49**, Suppl. 137 (Vessel structure studied by angiography and electron-microscopy etc.).
RAIMONDI, A. J., MULLAN, S. and EVANS, J. P. (1962) *J. Neurosurg.*, **19**, 731 (Ultrastructure).
RIDLEY, A. and CAVANAGH, J. B. (1971) *Brain*, **94**, 117 (Lymphocytic infiltration in gliomas).
RUBINSTEIN, L. J. (1956) *J. Path. Bact.*, **71**, 441 (Sarcoma arising in glioblastoma).
RUBINSTEIN, L. J. (1967) *J. Neurosurg.*, **26**, 542 (Extraneural metastases without previous surgery).
SWAEN, G. J. V., VOSSENAAR, T. and WYERS, H. J. G. (1964) *J. Path. Bact.*, **87**, 75 (Abnormal mitoses in malignant gliomas).

Plate 9. GLIOBLASTOMA MULTIFORME

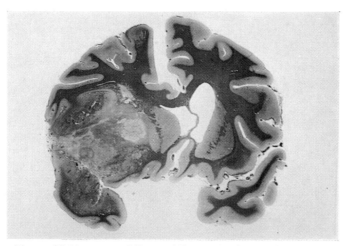

Fig. 1. Glioblastoma multiforme, filling much of the white matter of one cerebral hemisphere. There are many large necrotic zones within the tumour. Signs of cerebral swelling are present: the lateral ventricles are displaced and there is herniation of gyrus cinguli. (Celloidin PTAH × 0·5)

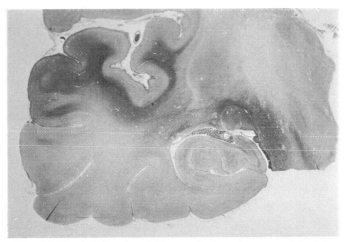

Fig. 2. Diffusely infiltrative glioblastoma in the white matter of the right temporal lobe is revealed in this section (by its dark appearance indicating hypercellularity). It was not suspected on naked-eye examination, and there was no displacement. (Celloidin Nissl   × 2)

GLIOBLASTOMA MULTIFORME
Case 8. Man aged 49

History. Three months' sudden attacks of dizziness and 'muddled thinking' each lasting a few minutes. Two weeks' severe early morning headache lasting twenty minutes to two hours, with nausea.

Examination. Bilateral papilloedema (worse on left). Nominal dysphasia (unable to name head of pin or winder of watch). Right facial weakness and right extensor plantar response.

Clinical diagnosis. Left temporal tumour.

Investigations. Carotid angiograms revealed a large anterior and middle temporal mass with no abnormal circulation.

Operation. Left temporal craniotomy. A pinkish-grey cystic tumour was found at the tip of the temporal lobe, about 3 cm in diameter, and a limited lobectomy was performed.

Follow-up. Immediate postoperative progress was good and after radiotherapy he returned to work (research in mathematics). One year later symptoms returned and he died shortly afterwards.

Microscopical appearances

A large part of the tumour is necrotic. The viable growth is characterized by hypercellularity, pleomorphism and vascular hyperplasia. There are cells of many varieties of shape and size; large, bizarre giant cells are conspicuous and among them mitotic figures are common. Glial fibres are sparse. There is dense collagenous connective tissue in relation to the prolific vessels. Lymphocytic cuffing is marked in the surrounding white matter.

Diagnosis. Glioblastoma multiforme.

Summary

This patient, distressed by the deterioration in his mental functions, was able to return to a high level of intellectual performance for a year following lobectomy and radiotherapy. At present, the effects of irradiation on malignant glial tumours of the astrocytoma–glioblastoma series can only be inferred: we do not know of any prospective study that establishes a significant difference between irradiated and non-irradiated subjects.

Marked perivascular lymphocytic cuffing is an interesting pathological finding in malignant gliomas and may point toward an active immune response (Ridley and Cavanagh 1971). In other respects the neoplasm is a typical glioblastoma.

Plate 10. GLIOBLASTOMA MULTIFORME

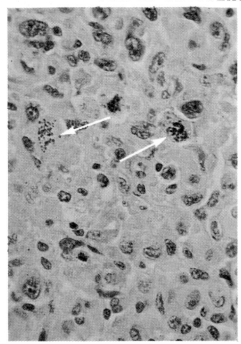

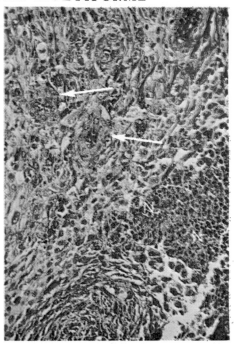

Fig. 1 (Case 8). The cells in this field have large oval nuclei with prominent nucleoli. Mitotic figures are common (arrows). (H & E   × 420)

Fig. 2 (Case 8). Pleomorphic cells, some with long processes arising at the poles of the cells, and hyperplastic capillaries (arrows). A portion of the tissue is necrotic (n). (PTAH   × 175)

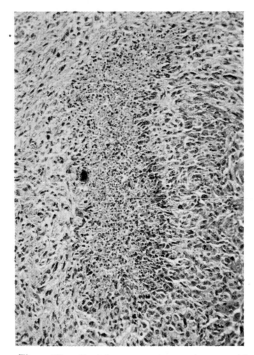

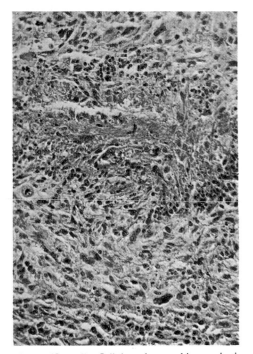

Fig. 3 (Case 8). A large central necrotic zone with surrounding palisade of cells with small darkly stained nuclei. (PTAH   × 105)

Fig. 4 (Case 8). Cellular pleomorphism, mitotic figures, focal necrosis and some glial fibres are all evident. (PTAH   × 175)

GLIOBLASTOMA MULTIFORME

Case 9. Woman aged 69

History. Five years previously, mastectomy for carcinoma. No local recurrence. Two weeks' confusion and difficulty with speech: visual disturbances on right.

Examination. Conscious and alert. Severe receptive and expressive dysphasia. Right homonymous hemianopia; early papilloedema left fundus; right pupil larger than left, reacting sluggishly. Limb reflexes abnormally brisk but equal, plantar responses flexor. Reduction of sensation to pinprick in right arm and right side of face. No sign of neoplasia on general examination.

Investigations. Scintiscan showed a left temporo-occipital lesion, confirmed by carotid angiogram. Left vertebral angiogram indicated the presence of an occipital mass extending to the temporal lobe with abnormal vessels.

Clinical diagnosis. Metastasis? Glioma?

Operation. Posterior parieto-occipital craniotomy. The cortex was flattened and pale. When incised a diffuse, friable, partly necrotic pink-grey tumour was encountered, merging with the brain. As much as possible of the growth was removed, down to the inferior surface of the lobe.

Follow-up. Immediate postoperative progress was good; the dysphasia improved. Two months later she died from recurrent growth.

Microscopical appearances

A highly cellular, pleomorphic tumour in which a pattern is formed of thick bundles of elongated spindle-shaped cells with numerous fine glial processes, alternating with groups of larger, mainly rounded cells with plentiful cytoplasm, large nuclei with prominent nucleoli but few glial fibres. There are some bizarre giant cells with abnormally large nuclei, and the incidence of mitosis is high. Large portions of the tumour are necrotic. There is extensive overgrowth of collagenous connective tissue related to hypertrophic blood vessels.

Diagnosis. Glioblastoma multiforme, giant cell type.

Summary

The history of a mastectomy suggested a metastatic tumour, but the sizeable lesion revealed by the angiogram looked more like a glioma. At operation the growth clearly merged with its surroundings.

The microscopical findings are of a tumour with great variation in cell morphology, deserving the term 'multiforme', and including giant cells of monstrous appearance.

Plate 11. GLIOBLASTOMA MULTIFORME

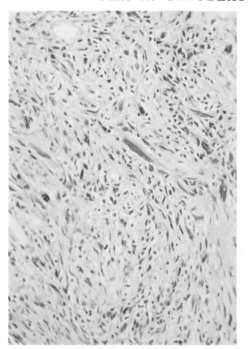

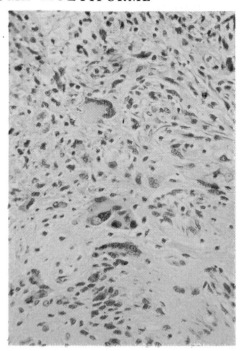

Fig. 1 (Case 9). Spindle-shaped cells of varied size and smaller cells with round nuclei make up this picture of a malignant glioma. A mitotic figure is present. (H & E   × 175)

Fig. 2 (Case 9). Another field of pleomorphic tumour. (H & E   × 210)

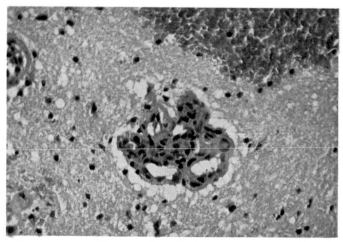

Fig. 3. A group of hyperplastic capillaries in the white matter beyond the confines of a glioblastoma. (H & E   × 265)

GLIOBLASTOMA–SARCOMA

Case 10. Man aged 53

History. Two months' tiredness and lack of energy. Four weeks' pain and numbness in the left side of the face, increasing sleepiness and deterioration in sense of direction: he would turn right instead of left and avoided using left hand.

Examination. Alert and well orientated but with impaired intellect; drawing a clockface was badly performed. Bilateral papilloedema, left homonymous hemianopia. Left facial and upper limb weakness, impaired position sense in left hand.

Investigations. Scintiscan indicated a deep posterotemporal lesion and this was confirmed by carotid angiograms.

Operation. Right temporoparietal craniotomy. The cortex was abnormal with pale expanded gyri. At 2 cm depth in the white matter, stringy, tough and, in part, soft diffuse tumour was encountered. Further dissection revealed a discrete tumour about the size of a walnut, thought to be a metastasis, and this was removed.

Follow-up. The patient continued to deteriorate and died from pneumonia one month after operation.

Microscopical appearances

A pleomorphic malignant tumour, portions of which are necrotic. Thick bands of connective tissue extend through the substance of the growth, producing a mottled appearance. Some of these bands are sparsely cellular and hyaline; others contain spindle fibroblasts and groups of undifferentiated malignant connective tissue tumour cells. Also within the connective tissue are groups of capillary blood vessels with abnormally prominent and prolific endothelial nuclei; some of these contain blood, but in others there is no lumen. The appearance of the prolific endothelial cells is often quite abnormal, with disorderly syncytial masses of oval nuclei and numerous mitotic figures. In contrast, the picture outside the connective tissue is that of a typical malignant glial tumour of mixed cell type: elongated perivascular cells with polar processes, gemistocytic astrocytes and cells resembling oligodendrocytes with round nuclei lying in a 'halo' of clear cytoplasm.

Diagnosis. Glioblastoma–sarcoma (malignant glioma with sarcomatous vascular proliferation).

Summary

The apparent demarcation of the tumour led the operator to the view that this was a metastasis. However, malignant gliomas are sometimes apparently circumscribed, especially when they infiltrate the leptomeninges and incorporate connective tissue into their substance. They can, indeed, mimic a meningioma.

Sarcomatous change in the vascular bed of a malignant glioma is a rare complication. It is much more common to find a necrotic glioma containing a large element of fibrovascular connective tissue, and the diagnosis depends upon the finding of unequivocal neoplasia in the vascular endothelium or associated fibroblasts.

Plate 12. GLIOSARCOMA

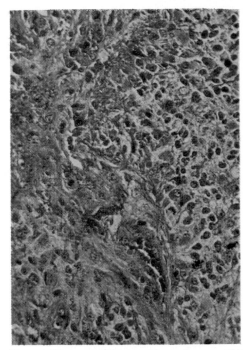

Fig. 1 (Case 10). Pleomorphic malignant glial tumour. Abnormal hyperplastic blood vessels are conspicuous. (PTAH × 265)

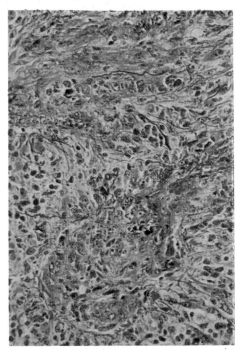

Fig. 2 (Case 10). Solid masses of prolific vascular tissue alternating with malignant glial tumour cells with numerous fine processes. (PTAH × 210)

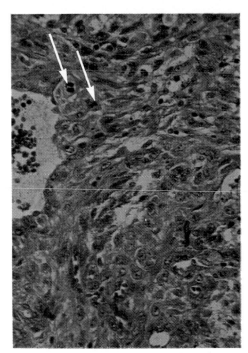

Fig. 3 (Case 10). A solid mass of neoplastic vascular tissue composed of cells with oval nuclei and prominent nucleoli with a high incidence of mitotic figures (arrows). The morphology is distinct from that of the glioblastoma and glial fibres are not present. (PTAH × 265)

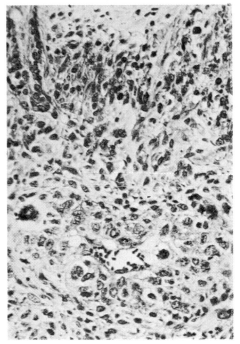

Fig. 4. In this case of glioblastoma–sarcoma only a few islands of glioma (PTAH-positive, reticulin-negative) remained. The bulk of the growth was sarcoma (PTAH-negative) (PTAH × 210)

OLIGODENDROGLIOMA

The oligodendroglioma (or oligodendrocytoma) is moderately common in the cerebral hemispheres and rare in the cerebellum and spinal cord. It is often considered to be a highly differentiated, slow-growing tumour, frequently calcified, and associated with a long history of symptoms. In a proportion of cases, however, the clinical course follows a more rapid tempo, and the cells are pleomorphic.

The classical appearance of these tumours has been recognized from the time of Bailey and Bucy's account (1929). The cells have large round nuclei, surrounded by a 'halo' of clear cytoplasm, and lie in a delicate honeycomb network of regular pattern (Plate 13, Fig. 1). Short straight or corkscrew-like processes can usually be demonstrated by PTAH or silver impregnation methods, but in a number of cases no processes are visible. The tissue is subdivided by thin-walled blood channels into pavement-like sections. Free-lying mucin is often present. A less common pattern of growth found in a proportion of oligo-dendrogliomas is of cells with slender, elongated nuclei arranged in parallel rows (see Plate 17, Fig. 4).

The less differentiated malignant (pleomorphic) tumours contain cells of irregular shape, with larger nuclei, coarsely granular chromatin and eosinophil cytoplasm; the well-ordered arrangement and clear 'haloes' are lost. The incidence of mitosis may be high. The blood vessels are thick-walled and prominent with endothelial hyperplasia approaching the degree typical of a glioblastoma. Glial cells of primitive astrocytic type, often with fine polar processes, may be arranged around the vessels (see Plate 18, Fig. 2) and when present in large numbers may result in the formation of a mixed glioma.

The final malignant picture of an oligodendroglioma may well be that of a growth whose cellular pleomorphism, necrosis and vascular changes invite the diagnosis of glioblastoma, and only the comparison of biopsy and subsequent necropsy material can then enable the evolution of the tumour to be appreciated.

Bibliography

BAILEY, P. and BUCY, P. C. (1929) *J. Path. Bact.*, **32,** 735 (The 'classic' report: detailed descriptions supplemented by metallic impregnations).

BARNARD, R. O. (1968) *J. Path. Bact.*, **96,** 113 (Malignancy: evolution toward glioblastoma).

BECK, DIANA J. K. and RUSSELL, DOROTHY S. (1942) *Brain*, **65,** 352 (Cerebrospinal spread; meningeal reaction).

EARNEST, F. III, KERNOHAN, J. W. and CRAIG, W. MCK. (1950) *Acta neurol. psychiat.*, **63,** 964 (Review of 200 cases).

LUSE, SARAH A. (1962) In *Biology and Treatment of Intracranial Tumors*, ed. W. S. Fields and P. C. Sharkey. Springfield, Ill.: Charles C Thomas (Ultrastructure).

RAVENS, J. R., ADAMKIEWICZ, L. L. and GROFF, R. A. (1955) *J. Neuropath. exp. Neurol.*, **14,** 142 (Mixed cytology demonstrated by metallic methods).

SMITH, BARBARA and BUTLER, MURIEL (1973) *Acta neuropath.*, **23,** 181 (Acid mucopolysaccharides in oligodendroglioma and Schwannoma).

ZÜLCH, K. J. (1965) See p. x.

Plate 13. OLIGODENDROGLIOMA

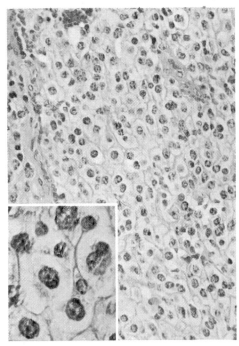

Fig. 1. Oligodendroglioma. The cells have large rounded nuclei surrounded by clear cytoplasm enclosed by well-defined membranes. (H & E × 265; H & E × approx. 1060)

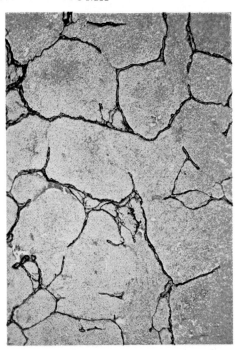

Fig. 2. Thin walled blood channels subdivide the tissue. (Reticulin × 26)

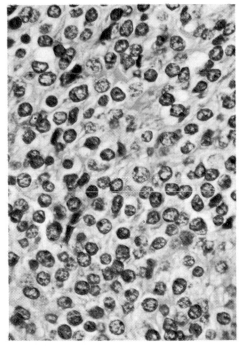

Fig. 3. In this oligodendroglioma the nuclei are larger, more closely packed, and less regular in shape. (PAS × 420)

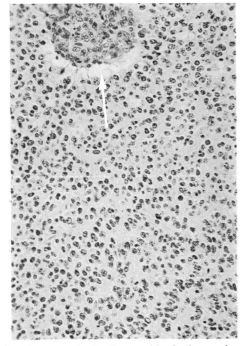

Fig. 4. Oligodendroglioma with focal vascular proliferation resulting in a mass of endothelial cells (arrow). (H & E × 210)

OLIGODENDROGLIOMA

Case 11. Woman aged 44

History. One year increasingly forgetful of recent events. Six months' severe bifrontal head-aches, worse in the morning, for one month associated with nausea. Two months' epileptic attacks with loss of consciousness, jactitation of all four limbs and occasional incontinence.

Examination. Euphoric and fatuous; easily distracted. Mild bilateral papilloedema. Right upper motor neuron facial weakness.

Investigations. Skull radiograph showed erosion of dorsum sellae. Scintiscan: no abnormal uptake. Carotid angiogram revealed a left frontal tumour with abnormal circulation extending across the genu of the corpus callosum. The appearances were confirmed by ventriculogram.

Operation. Left frontal craniotomy showed the frontal lobe largely replaced by tumour with a mottled red colour presenting in the middle frontal convolution 2 cm behind the frontal pole. Frontal lobectomy extending to the genu was carried out. The incision passed across the tumour and the remaining posterior portion was removed separately.

Follow-up. Following surgery and a course of radiotherapy remained well for two and a half years when the tumour recurred. She died three and a half years postoperatively.

Microscopical appearances

The tumour is composed of cells with large round vesicular nuclei of regular shape. Mitotic figures are few. Often, the nuclei lie free in a zone of apparently clear cytoplasm, giving rise to the characteristic 'honeycomb' appearance. Blood vessels are slender and thin-walled; there are a number of small focal haemorrhages. The edge of the growth has no well-defined margin and where there is infiltration into the surrounding white matter there are numerous foci of calcification. The tumour has also spread widely under the pia mater, in places infiltrating the outer laminae of the cortex.

Diagnosis. Typical oligodendroglioma.

Summary

The onset of symptoms in this patient was gradual, building up progressively in the last months before admission. The calcification of the tumour, evident microscopically, was not sufficient to be visible in the skull radiographs, unlike many cases in which the presence of an oligodendroglioma can be suspected from the appearances of the skull pictures.

The pathological finding of a 'typical' oligodendroglioma is often associated with a slow evolution of symptoms, but there is great individual variation. This tumour was not examined *post mortem* and it may be that it developed a more malignant character.

Plate 14. OLIGODENDROGLIOMA

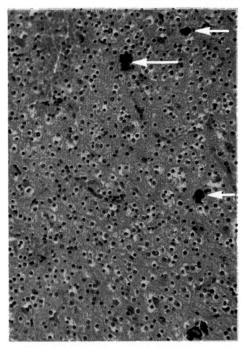

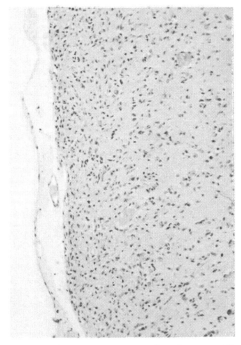

Fig. 1 (Case 11). Typical oligodendroglioma with focal calcification of the tumour tissue (arrows) and haemorrhage. (H & E   × 175)

Fig. 2 (Case 11). Subpial aggregation of tumour cells infiltrating the cortex away from the main mass. (H & E   × 130)

OLIGODENDROGLIOMA

Case 12. Man aged 44

History. Seven years' left-sided focal epileptic fits, up to two per day, involving the face, arm and leg. Four years' *grand mal* fits, four attacks in all, controlled with drugs. Two years' progressive weakness of the left leg and loss of position sense in left leg and left arm, transiently worse after each focal attack. Few days' right-sided headache in the early morning.

Examination. Very mild left hemiparesis, including face, more marked in the leg. Impaired joint position sense in left leg.

Investigations. Skull radiograph revealed spotty calcification in the right parietal lobe. Right carotid angiogram showed a parietal tumour deeply situated but extending close to the surface on the medial side.

Operation. Right parieto-occipital craniotomy. The cortex was bulging, but no tumour presented on the surface. Needle aspiration yielded purple tumour tissue and via a small incision large quantities of glioma were sucked out from the white matter.

Follow-up. After a course of radiotherapy he made a steady improvement. One year later only minimal signs of left-sided weakness remained and he had no complaints.

Microscopical appearances

The tumour consists of cells with large round or oval nuclei, a coarse chromatin network, one or more prominent nucleoli and varied amounts of eosinophil cytoplasm. The incidence of mitotic figures is moderately high. Less common are the typical cells of an oligodendroglioma with round uniform nuclei sometimes with a clear cytoplasmic halo. In many places the pattern of the growth is typical oligodendroglioma, with thin-walled capillaries subdividing the cells into small groups. Elsewhere there are long parallel rows of cells and some perivascular 'pseudo-rosettes'. There is frequent 'droplet' calcification of the tumour tissue and of its gliotic edges.

Diagnosis. Oligodendroglioma with atypical pattern.

Summary

Treatment of this tumour produced a very satisfactory result, despite the variation in microscopical appearances and the presence of mitotic figures. In a study of a large series of cases Earnest et al. (1950) found that no correlation could be made between the presence of mitotic figures in an oligodendroglioma and the prognosis.

The arrangement of the cells in parallel rows and pseudorosettes is a recognized, though less common, variation of the usual pattern. Astrocytic cells were not found in this tumour.

Plate 15. OLIGODENDROGLIOMA

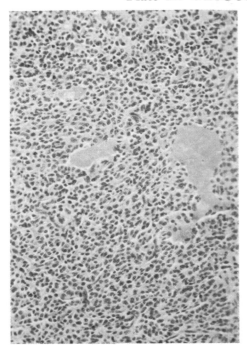 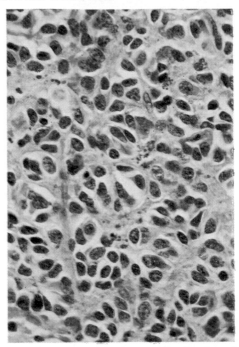

Fig. 1 (Case 12). Oligodendroglioma composed of cells of more varied appearance than the preceding examples. Many cells have eosinophil cytoplasm and the clear haloes are less conspicuous. There is no vascular hyperplasia. (H & E   × 175)

Fig. 2 (Case 12). At higher magnification the cell nuclei are oval or pyriform with coarsely granular chromatin. (H & E   × 420)

OLIGODENDROGLIOMA

Case 13. Woman aged 39

History. Six years' epilepsy initially consisting of attacks of numbness in the fingers of the left hand. One year later major attacks developed with unconsciousness and jactitations of the left side of the body, occurring about twice a week. Weakness of left arm appeared about the same time. A diagnosis of calcifying glioma in right frontoparietal region was made (on the basis of skull radiographs) one year after onset of attacks. Surgery not advised at that time in view of location in the motor radiation since a more severe paresis would have resulted. After five years of reasonably normal life, nine months' progressive hemiplegia with intellectual impairment and deterioration in memory with emotional lability occurred.

Examination. Dementia. Bilateral papilloedema. Left hemiplegia. Impaired joint-position sense in left hand.

Investigations. Skull radiograph: mottled calcification in the right parietal area had not increased in size. Erosion of dorsum sellae. Arteriogram revealed a very large tumour extending deeply without neoplastic circulation.

Operation. Parietal craniotomy. Red-grey tumour presented through the centre of the motor area, extending deeply into the hemisphere, infiltrating brain tissue. Partial removal carried out to relieve intracranial tension.

Follow-up. The patient died two days later of severe cerebral oedema.

Microscopical appearances

In the cortex there are circumscribed nodules of tumour of fairly regular pattern; the cells have small round vesicular nuclei separated by faintly staining cytoplasm from the cell margins. Near the periphery there are foci of concentric calcification. Several of the numerous thin-walled blood vessels have ruptured, giving rise to haemorrhage. The tumour has also extended through the white matter and here the cell type is much more varied; the nuclei tend to be larger, with coarsely granular chromatin and prominent nucleoli; mitotic figures are common.

Diagnosis. Oligodendroglioma (with transition to malignant type).

Summary

This patient's illness proceeded in two distinct phases. At first there were left-sided epileptic fits that did not change over the course of years, and did not interfere with the patient's normal life. A calcified glioma was found, but operative removal not attempted. Five years later the second phase began. The patient deteriorated rapidly with dementia and left hemiplegia.

The pathological findings are in accord. A circumscribed, calcified oligodendroglioma of typical cell-type occupies the position of the lesion visible on the skull radiographs. Around it a diffusely infiltrative neoplasm of pleomorphic type extends deeply into the white matter.

Plate 16. OLIGODENDROGLIOMA

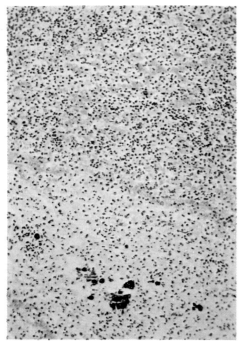

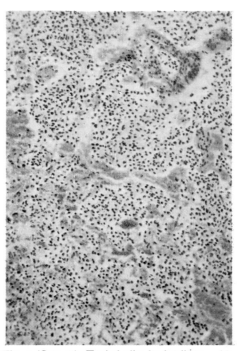

Fig. 1 (Case 13). There are numerous haemorrhages into the tumour. At the periphery of the growth the tissues are calcified. (H & E   × 105)

Fig. 2 (Case 13). Typical oligodendroglioma, with haemorrhages from overdistended capillaries. (H & E × 105)

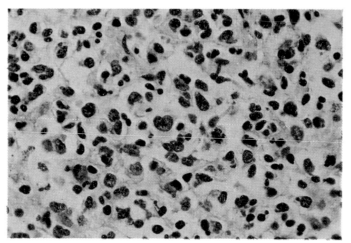

Fig. 3 (Case 13). In this field the tumour cells are of much more varied size and shape: mitotic figures are present. (H & E   × 420)

OLIGODENDROGLIOMA
Case 14. Woman aged 47

History. Two weeks' fits. The first attack followed a severe headache with convulsions starting in the right side of the face and then becoming generalized. One day later she was admitted to hospital in status epilepticus and controlled with phenytoin and phenobarbitone.

Examination. Alert but irritable. Right spastic hemiparesis.

Investigations. Left carotid angiogram indicated the presence of a frontal tumour. Scintiscan showed increased uptake low in the frontal region.

Clinical diagnosis. Glioma or metastasis in left frontal lobe. Meningioma less likely.

Operation. Left frontal craniotomy. Greyish-white infiltrative tumour presented through the cortex and extended back as a large mass overlying the Sylvian fissure in the post-frontal zone. A partial removal was carried out, keeping within the confines of the tumour.

Follow-up. Following radiotherapy she complained of vomiting. She was free of fits until nine months later when she deteriorated with a presumed recurrent tumour.

Microscopical appearances

Some parts of this tumour are typical oligodendroglioma: the cells have large, uniform, round nuclei lying in clear cytoplasm in a well-defined network. In many places, however, there is an abrupt transition to cells characterized by larger nuclei of irregular outline that tend to be arranged in parallel rows, or to be orientated round blood vessels. Among the latter cell-type, mitotic figures are relatively common.

PTAH staining demonstrates that there are occasional cells of the astrocytic series scattered in the tumour, but that both the chief cell-types are oligodendrocytic. The numerous blood vessels are mostly thin-walled channels and there is no endothelial hyperplasia. At the periphery of the growth there is abundant calcification.

Diagnosis. Oligodendroglioma with an unusual pattern of growth.

Summary

The microscopical appearances of this tumour are, in part, those of a typical oligodendroglioma and, in part, those of a growth of cells of less regular appearance with larger nuclei tending to be orientated around blood vessels or to be arranged in parallel columns. The cells are still, clearly, of oligodendrocytic type, and astrocytes are sparse.

This morphological variation and the presence of numerous mitotic figures suggested a rapid tempo of growth and since total removal of the tumour was not possible, recurrence was to be expected.

Plate 17. OLIGODENDROGLIOMA

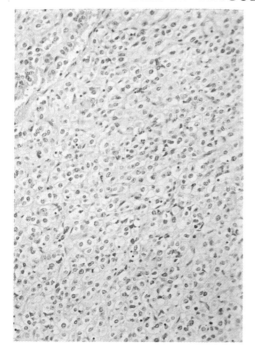

Fig. 1 (Case 14). Typical oligodendroglioma. (H & E × 130)

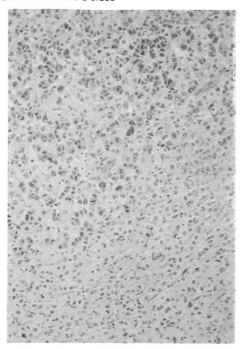

Fig. 2 (Case 14). There is a transition from typical oligodendroglioma to a growth of larger cells with a higher mitotic incidence. (H & E × 130)

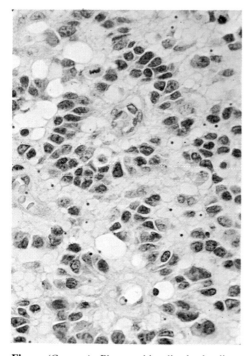

Fig. 3 (Case 14). Pleomorphic oligodendroglioma cells clustered around small blood vessels. (H & E × 530)

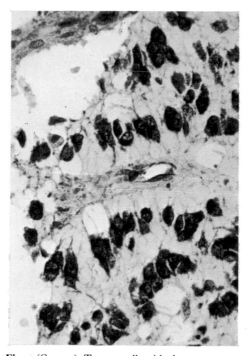

Fig. 4 (Case 14). Tumour cells with short processes arranged in parallel perivascular rows. (PTAH × 530)

OLIGODENDROGLIOMA–ASTROCYTOMA

Case 15. Man aged 45

History. Five months' change in personality: apathetic, inert and would stare into space. Headaches intermittently, usually in morning, associated with nausea. Two months' increasing dysphasia. Two convulsions started on left side and became generalized with loss of consciousness.

Examination. Accessible, with receptive and expressive dysphasia, particularly the former. Difficulty in cooperating. Early bilateral papilloedema. Mild left hemiparesis with increased reflexes in arm and leg and extensor plantar response.

Investigations. Carotid angiograms disclosed large bifrontal masses, probably involving the genu of the corpus callosum. No neoplastic circulation.

Operation. Left frontal craniotomy. Hard tumour presented on the surface over 6×5 cm in the posterior frontal area. Near the surface the tumour was well demarcated, but deeply it merged into the surrounding white matter. A palliative partial removal was carried out.

Follow-up. Patient died seven days postoperatively.

Necropsy. The brain was swollen. Blood clot and 'gelfoam' occupied the operative site in the left frontal lobe. The genu of the corpus callosum was greatly thickened with tumour tissue and the right frontal lobe contained grey gelatinous tumour flecked with haemorrhage covering approximately $5 \times 2 \times 2$ cm.

Microscopical appearances

A portion of the left frontal tumour is a typical calcified oligodendroglioma with rounded nuclei and 'clear' cytoplasm. In the corpus callosum and right hemisphere the growth is much more varied, with many cells of the astrocyte series including bipolar cells, with elongated processes radiating from around blood vessels.

Diagnosis. Mixed glioma with oligodendrocytic and astrocytic elements.

Summary

This was an example of a 'butterfly' glioma involving both frontal lobes and the genu of the corpus callosum. In the left frontal lobe the growth is typical oligodendroglioma, calcified near its margins. Elsewhere the tumour is much more varied and astrocytic cells predominate. The appearances in the corpus callosum are of a pure malignant astrocytoma.

Plate 18. OLIGODENDROGLIOMA

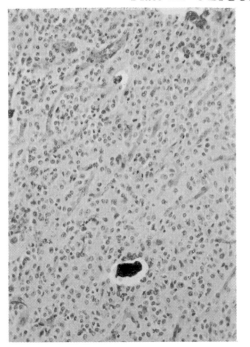

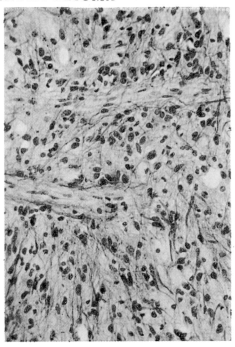

Fig. 1 (Case 15). Typical oligodendroglioma with focal calcification. There are numerous straight capillaries. (H & E   × 175)

Fig. 2 (Case 15). Cells of the astrocyte series radiate from the walls of small blood vessels. (PTAH × 210)

EPENDYMOMA

Ependymomas are composed of differentiated ependymal cells and may arise in relation to any part of the ventricular system. They are specially common in the fourth ventricle, less common in the lateral or third ventricles and make up a high proportion (over 60 per cent) of the intramedullary gliomas of the spinal cord, where syringomyelic cavitation may sometimes be associated.

The cells resemble normal ependyma to a greater or lesser degree. They tend to form clusters or 'rosettes' (*see below*), around a small lumen, or tubules. Under some conditions, the tumour cells develop long fibrillary processes, just as normal ependymal cells may, when they cease to line the surface of a cavity. A common grouping is the perivascular *pseudorosette* in which the cells are orientated towards blood vessels, and sometimes they radiate from around the vessels with a 'sun-ray' appearance. Some examples (the 'papillary' or 'trabecular' ependymomas) have a well-formed papillary structure that may closely resemble that of the choroid plexus papilloma. The *myxopapillary* ependymoma is a special type containing quantities of mucoid connective tissue and is found exclusively in the region of the cauda equina; the microscopical structure recalls that of the filum terminale.

One characteristic of both ependymoma cells and normal ependyma is the possession of *blepharoplasts*, tiny rod-shaped bodies tending to be clustered close to the nucleus and recognizable only in PTAH-stained sections at high powers of magnification. In biopsy material, due to their similarity to mitochondria, they may be impossible to identify. Electron microscopical study (Brightman and Palay 1963) has demonstrated that blepharoplasts correspond to the basal bodies at the terminations of the cilia normally present in mature ependymal cells.

Rosettes

Considerable confusion exists over the significance implied in this term which has been used for certain different types of structure found in different tumours. In ependymoma (and ependymoblastoma) the cells may be grouped around a small central lumen to form a true *ependymal* rosette. These are usually less common than the perivascular pseudo-rosettes mentioned already. In medulloblastoma and neuroblastoma, rosettes ('Homer Wright rosettes') are also found, but with no lumen or blood vessel at the centre of the cell-grouping. In retinoblastoma, Flexner–Wintersteiner rosettes with lumens are characteristic. In pineocytoma another type of 'rosette' is formed by the arrangement of cells around an oval faintly eosinophil zone that appears structureless in H & E stained sections (*see* Plate 59, Fig. 1) but which may contain argyrophilic fibrils if appropriate metallic methods are used.

SUBEPENDYMOMA

The ependymal cells normally lie on a bed of neuroglial tissue, which naturally is capable of proliferation, and the name subependymoma is used for mixed tumours in which cells of ependymal type are intimately associated with extensive overgrowth of fibrillary glia (*see* Plate 23, Figs 1–3).

Plate 19. EPENDYMOMA

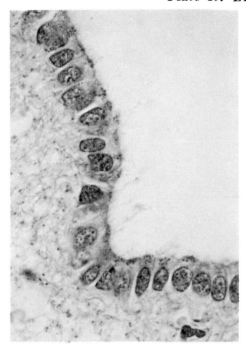

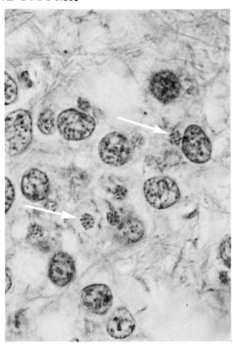

Fig. 1. Blepharoplasts clustered at the free margins of ependymal epithelial cells. (PTAH × 1190)

Fig. 2. Clusters of blepharoplasts (arrows) in ependymoma cells. (PTAH × 1590)

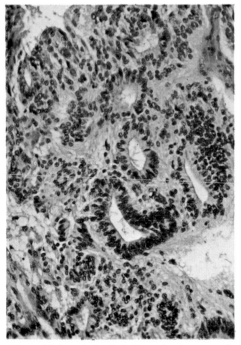

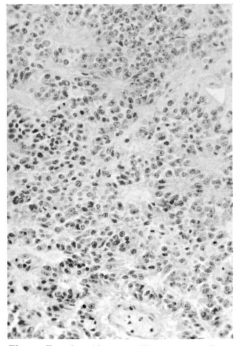

Fig. 3. Well marked tubule formation in an ependymoma. (H & E × 105)

Fig. 4. Ependymoblastoma. The tumour cells are of more primitive type than those of a typical ependymoma and mitotic figures are present. There are well-formed rosettes. (H & E × 210)

EPENDYMOBLASTOMA

This term, which has been used rather indiscriminately for poorly differentiated ependymoma, has recently been carefully defined by Rubinstein (1970). It can be applied to certain rare malignant tumours of early childhood composed, appropriately, of primitive cells, but with well-marked ependymal rosette formation. Cells in mitosis are numerous and may be found in the rosettes.

CHOROID PLEXUS PAPILLOMA

The papillary tumours of the choroid plexus affect the fourth, lateral and third ventricles in that order of frequency. Microscopically these growths closely resemble normal choroid plexus and consist in a proliferation of columnar epithelium usually in the form of a single layer of cells mounted on a fibrovascular stalk to form a papillary process (*see* Plate 24, Fig. 1). Unlike the papillary ependymoma, however, the vascular stroma does not contain glial tissue. Malignant changes ('choroid plexus carcinoma') are rare (Lewis 1967).

COLLOID CYST

Colloid cysts of the third ventricle are rare (*see* Plate 25, Figs 1–2). If small, they may be asymptomatic, while the larger cysts may produce intermittent attacks of acute hydrocephalus. The origin of these cysts has provoked discussion: some are believed to develop from the paraphysis cerebri, but many are probably of ependymal origin (Ariëns Kappers 1955) and for this reason they are included in this section. Their appearance and behaviour suggest a maldevelopmental lesion rather than a true tumour.

Bibliography

BRIGHTMAN, M. W. and PALAY, S. L. (1963) *J. Cell Biol.*, **19**, 415.
FRENCH, J. D. and BUCY, P. C. (1948) *J. Neurosurg.*, **5**, 433 (Subependymoma of septum pellucidum).
FOKES, E. C., jun. and EARLE, K. M. (1969) *J. Neurosurg.*, **30**, 585 (180 cases surveyed).
GOEBEL, H. H. and CRAVIOTO, H. (1972) *J. Neuropath. exp. Neurol.*, **31**, 54 (Ultrastructure of human and experimental ependymomas).
POSER, C. M. (1956) *The Relationship between Syringomyelia and Neoplasm.* Springfield, Ill.: Charles C Thomas.
QUEIROZ, L. S., LOPES DE FARIA, J. and CRUZNETO, J. N. (1975) *J. Path. Bact.*, **115**, 207 (Pontine ependymoblastoma).
RINGERTZ, N. and REYMOND, A. (1949) *J. Neuropath. exp. Neurol.*, **8**, 355 (Series of seventy-two ependymomas).
RUBINSTEIN, L. J. (1970) *Arch. Path.*, **90**, 35 (Ependymoblastoma).
SLOOFF, J. L., KERNOHAN, J. W. and MACCARTY, C. S. (1964) See p. x.

Choroid plexus papilloma

LEWIS, P. (1967) *Brain*, **90**, 177 (Malignant choroid plexus tumour).
MATSON, D. D. and CROFTON, F. D. L. (1960) *J. Neurosurg.*, **17**, 1002 (Choroid plexus papilloma in childhood).
MORELLO, G. and MIGLIAVACCA, F. (1964) *J. Neurol. Neurosurg. Psychiat.*, **27**, 445 (Choroid papillomas in the cerebellopontine angle).
SMITH, J. F. (1955) *J. Neuropath. exp. Neurol.*, **14**, 442 (Association with hydrocephalus).

Colloid cyst

ARIENS KAPPERS, J. (1955) *J. comp. Neurol.*, **102**, 425 (Origin of cyst).
KELLY, R. (1951) *Brain*, **74**, 23.

EPENDYMOMA
Case 16. Girl aged 18

History. Seven weeks' throbbing headache over the left eye. It spread to the whole of the left side of the scalp, usually worse in the morning, lasted four to twelve hours and occurred every two to five days. Five weeks' double vision on looking to the left and difficulty using the left hand. In four weeks, three episodes of vomiting.

Examination. Marked bilateral papilloedema. Slight ataxia of right hand. Right hemiparesis.

Investigations. Carotid angiogram disclosed a left frontoparietal mass with no pathological circulation.

Operation. Left frontal craniotomy. The motor and pre-motor cortex were broadened to a width of 4 cm across with red-grey friable tumour sprouting onto the surface. A large cyst was drained of 40 ml of fluid but only the superficial part of the neoplasm could be removed.

Follow-up. The initial pathological report suggested metastatic carcinoma, but no primary was found after thorough investigation. One year later the tumour recurred. At second operation large portions of the growth were removed from a recurrence anterior to the previous operative site. After two more years she was given radiotherapy for a second recurrence. Five years after the first operation the patient suffered bilateral visual deterioration and frontal lobectomy was performed, followed by further radiotherapy. She died eight years from the onset of symptoms.

Microscopical appearances

The tumour is composed of solid and papillary masses of well-defined polygonal cells with tubules of varying diameter, lined by cuboidal, occasionally ciliated, cells. Mucin is present with the tubules. Mitoses are not present.

Diagnosis. Ependymoma (tubular and papillary).

Summary

In this case the diagnosis of metastatic adenocarcinoma was suggested by the pathologist on the basis of a tumour with mucin-filled tubules lined by epithelial cells. This is a potential pitfall if the appearances of an ependymoma are not borne in mind. The course of the illness and its subsequent progress, with multiple recurrences becoming difficult to control either by surgery or radiotherapy, is quite typical of a relatively well-differentiated glioma.

Plate 20. EPENDYMOMA

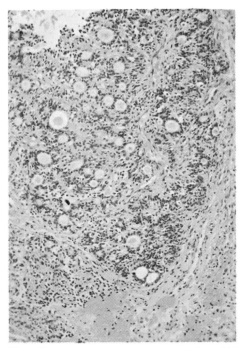

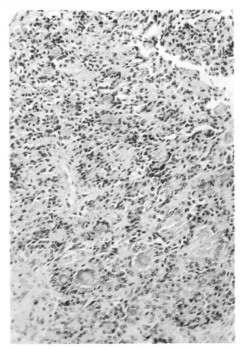

Fig. 1 (Case 16). Ependymoma composed of cuboidal and polyhedral cells with numerous tubules. (H & E × 105)

Fig. 2 (Case 16). Mucin is contained within some of the tubules. (Alcian blue × 105)

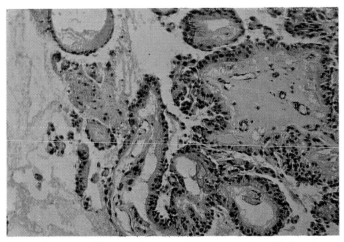

Fig. 3. A myxopapillary ependymoma of the cauda equina with abundant mucin. (Alcian blue × 105)

EPENDYMOMA

Case 17. Man aged 60

History. Two years' left-sided sciatica. Attacks of pain 'like burning oil' began in the buttocks passing down the back of the left leg to the foot. The pain increased with coughing, straining or movement and was worse at night. Frequency of micturition and nocturia for several years.

Examination. Marked limitation of lumbar movement; straight-leg raising 50° right, 45° left; severely impaired pain sensation in the first left sacral dermatome S1; mild impairment of S2–3 and right L5, with increased sensitivity to pain left L5. There was 2·5 cm wasting of left thigh muscles. Bilateral weakness of dorsiflexion of ankles and extensor halluces longi.

Investigations. Myelogram revealed a rounded intrathecal lesion at the level of L2–3, with a complete block.

Clinical diagnosis. Neurofibroma of left L5 root or ependymoma of filum terminale.

Operation. Lumbar laminectomy. On opening the dura a plum-red tumour 3 cm long was exposed attached to the filum terminale with the roots of the cauda equina splayed round it. The tumour was excised with the filum without disrupting the tenuous capsule.

Follow-up. Six years later the patient was well, with no disability.

Microscopical appearances

The tumour is composed of well-defined polygonal or columnar cells with very regular oval nuclei arranged either in papillae about a central core of hyaline tissue containing blood vessels, or in tubular formation, or in compact cellular masses separated by delicate vascularized stroma. Mitotic figures are not a feature.

Diagnosis. Papillary ependymoma of the filum terminale.

Summary

The lumbosacral region is a fairly common site for an ependymoma and the myxopapillary type of ependymoma is most common in this region. The tumour was contained within a distinct capsule and after removal did not recur. The possibility of a neurofibroma had been considered up to the time of operative exposure when it became clear that this tumour was attached to the filum.

Plate 21. EPENDYMOMA

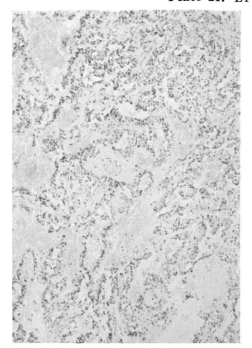

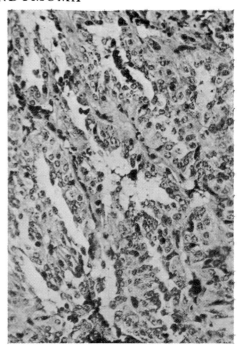

Fig. 1 (Case 17). Ependymoma with a well-defined papillary pattern. There are small haemorrhages. (H & E × 105)

Fig. 2. Polygonal cells with regular oval vesicular nuclei. Some cells are angulated towards the lumen of a blood vessel. (PTAH × 265)

EPENDYMOMA
Case 18. Man aged 50

History. Nine years' pain in the neck and between both shoulder-blades, subsequently spreading down both arms into the tips of the fingers, worse on the left side than the right, and most severe early in the morning. For six years pain persisted without progression, then for six months pain more severe, difficulty in swallowing, arms weaker, legs stiff, frequency of micturition.

Examination. Mentally normal. Right Horner's syndrome. Right ptosis. Left palatal and vocal cord paresis. Left sternomastoid weak and wasted. Fibrillation of tongue. Wasting and fibrillation of shoulder girdle and arm muscles bilaterally; severe wasting of small hand muscles. Finger-to-nose ataxia. Left knee and ankle jerks increased; both plantar responses extensor. Loss of sensation to pain and temperature over the left side of the face, neck, upper limbs and trunk down to D5 segmental level and over the left side of the face. Position sensation impaired in both upper limbs. Gait spastic and ataxic.

Investigations. Lumbar myelogram showed diffuse expansion of the spinal cord from C1 to C7 vertebrae.

Clinical diagnosis. Probably intramedullary tumour, possibly syringomyelia. In view of the danger of increasing swallowing difficulties by operative decompression no surgery was advised and a course of radiotherapy given.

Follow-up. Immediate but temporary improvement. Two years later pain became severe again; large doses of analgesics required. He developed further wasting of muscles in the upper limbs and spastic paraparesis and sensory loss extending down to D8 level, but survived for three more years.

Necropsy. Solid, grey-white intramedullary tumour occupied 3 cm length of the upper cervical cord. Below the tumour there was a syringomyelic cavity with surrounding softening extending through the lower cervical segments to D1. Above the tumour another syrinx extended through the medulla almost to the obex. No abnormality rostral to the pons.

Microscopical appearances

Upper cervical. The cord is almost completely replaced by a well-differentiated ependymoma composed of cells of regular size with oval, vesicular nuclei. The cells tend to be arranged in radiating cords and in pseudo-rosettes around the numerous blood channels. Blepharoplasts are prominent in many tumour cells. Mitotic figures are rare. There is pigment in macrophages indicating old haemorrhage.

Low cervical. Two syringomyelic cavities are present, each is surrounded by astrocytic gliosis with Rosenthal fibres. A nest of ependymal cells, having prominent blepharoplasts, is present in the commissural region separate from the cavities.

Diagnosis. Ependymoma, syringomyelia.

Summary

Ependymomas may arise at any level of the spinal cord and in this case, in addition to the tumour, syringomyelic cavities extended in a caudal direction to D1, and rostrally into the medulla. Cavitation of this kind is a recognized complication of ependymoma, astrocytoma, dermoid cyst and haemangioblastoma of the cord (Poser 1956).

Plate 22. EPENDYMOMA

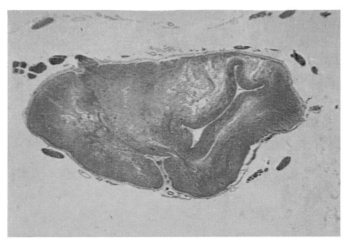

Fig. 1 (Case 18). Syrinx in cervical cord. (H & E and Luxol Fast Blue × 4)

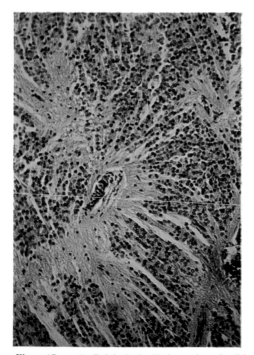

Fig. 2 (Case 18). Polyhedral cells in cords and solid masses tending to form a radial pattern around blood vessels. (PTAH × 130)

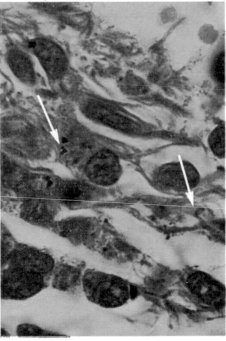

Fig. 3 (Case 18). Blepharoplasts (arrows) in ependymoma cells. (PTAH × 1325)

SUBEPENDYMOMA
Case 19. Woman aged 30

History. Ten days' headache affecting left side and also back of the neck. Four days' episodes of severe headache with weakness and unsteadiness followed by vomiting and photophobia.

Examination. Mentally normal but lethargic and pyrexial. Mild neck stiffness. Fine nystagmus on extremes of lateral gaze. Tendon reflexes increased on the right with right plantar equivocal.

Investigations. Cerebrospinal fluid: protein 140 mg/100 ml xanthochromic. Scintiscan normal. Carotid angiogram: no aneurysm or other abnormality. Vertebral angiogram suggestive of mass in fourth ventricle. Air encephalogram: air failed to enter ventricular system. Ventriculogram (using Myodil), indicated an intrinsic fourth ventricular tumour.

Operation. Midline posterior fossa exploration. Grey tumour, approximately 3 cm in diameter, occupied the whole of the lower half of the fourth ventricle and protruded out to separate the cerebellar tonsils. The tumour contained a cavity filled with old blood clot. It was removed completely except for a small zone infiltrating into the brain stem close to the superior cerebellar peduncle.

Follow-up. Improved and two months later was leading a normal life.

Microscopical appearances

The tumour tissue is sparsely cellular and consists of a dense matrix of glial fibres containing scattered groups of cells with large vesicular nuclei that resemble ependymal epithelia. In a few places the tissue is calcified.

Diagnosis. Subependymoma.

Summary

The short history of headache, becoming more and more severe, the associated vomiting and the findings of nystagmus, right hemiparesis and neck stiffness were all quite compatible with a posterior fossa tumour, but the possibility of a leaking aneurysm of the circle of Willis had to be considered and excluded by angiography. The diagnosis was indicated by ventriculogram and established at operation.

The subependymoma is a slow-growing, fairly uncommon, glioma, consisting of groups of ependymal cells in a dense astroglial matrix. It may be asymptomatic and be discovered as a chance finding *post mortem*.

Plate 23. SUBEPENDYMOMA

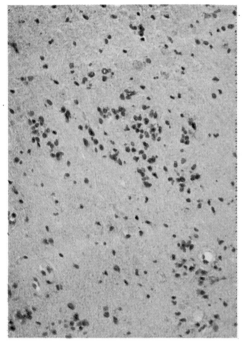

Fig. 1 (Case 19). Isolated clusters of cells of ependymal type in an eosinophil matrix. (H & E × 175)

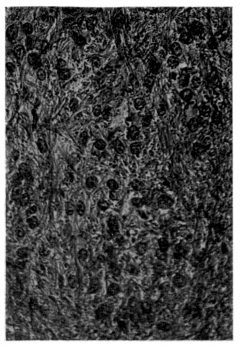

Fig. 2 (Case 19). Ependymal cells with oval vesicular nuclei and prominent nucleoli amidst numerous glial fibrils. (PTAH × 400)

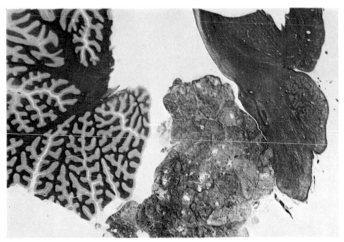

Fig. 3. Growth filling the fourth ventricle and herniating between the cerebellar tonsils. (PTAH × 1·6)

CHOROID PLEXUS PAPILLOMA

Case 20. Woman aged 42

History. Six months' 'giddy spells' and occipital headache, worse in the early morning, and associated with slight neck stiffness. Each headache was sharp and spasmodic, lasting about thirty seconds. For five days headache more severe. Collapsed in street as a result of legs giving way without loss of consciousness and was admitted to hospital.

Examination. Bilateral papilloedema; nystagmus coarse and slow on looking to the right. Mild hypertonia in all limbs but with bilateral cerebellar ataxia more marked on the right.

Clinical diagnosis. Posterior fossa tumour.

Investigations. Electroencephalogram disclosed severe abnormalities compatible with a posterior fossa tumour. Ventriculogram showed a large mass in the fourth ventricle on the right side.

Operation. Posterior fossa exploration. A large purple-grey firm tumour was found forming the right lateral wall of the fourth ventricle. The bulk of the growth was removed but a portion had to be left because of its close relationship to the nuclei of the ninth, tenth and eleventh cranial nerves.

Follow-up. The patient recovered consciousness but suddenly developed respiratory arrest and died six hours after the operation. At necropsy a large fresh blood clot was found.

Microscopical appearances

The tumour has a regular, almost uniform, structure of papillary processes lined by columnar cells with oval vesicular nuclei. Each group of processes has a central fibrovascular core.

Diagnosis. Choroid plexus papilloma.

Summary

The presenting symptoms and signs strongly indicated a tumour in the posterior fossa, and this was localized to the fourth ventricle by the ventriculogram. Ependymoma, subependymoma and choroid plexus papilloma were all possibilities to be considered. The most common situation for a papilloma of the choroid is in the fourth ventricle.

These tumours are commonly benign and amenable to operative removal, but their vascularity may lead, as in this case, to complicating haemorrhage.

Plate 24. CHOROID PLEXUS PAPILLOMA

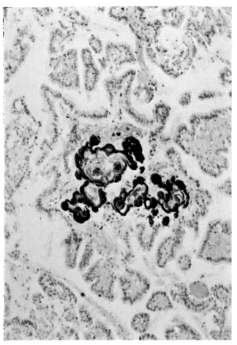

Fig. 1 (Case 20). Focal calcification of the papillary tumour. There is a close resemblance to normal choroid plexus. (H & E   × 175)

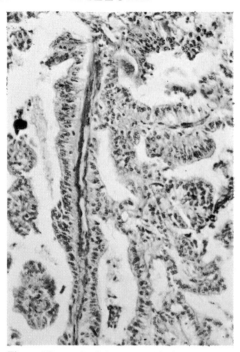

Fig. 2 (Case 20). Columnar epithelial cells lining the papillae. (PTAH   × 175)

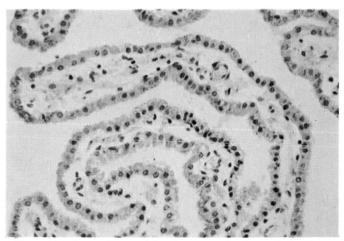

Fig. 3. Another papilloma with cells of low columnar and ciliated type in a month-old baby. (H & E   × 210)

COLLOID CYST
Case 21. Woman aged 46

History. Six months' almost daily attacks of severe headache, beginning behind both eyes and radiating round the skull to the back of the neck. Each attack lasted several hours and was relieved by lying down. Occasional vomiting. Five months' sudden falls without warning and without loss of consciousness, but always after the onset of the headache.

Examination. Memory poor; other mental functions normal. Bilateral papilloedema.

Investigations. Carotid angiogram indicated marked dilatation of the lateral ventricles. Ventriculography confirmed the hydrocephalus and showed occlusion of the foramen of Monro by a smooth mass projecting upwards from the posterior lip of the foramen.

Operation. Right frontal craniotomy. A firm, rounded pink-yellow tumour was obstructing the greatly dilated foramen of Monro. Numerous tiny arteries ran to the tumour from the right and left choroid plexuses. Firm creamy material was aspirated from it and the tumour capsule dissected from the margins of the foramen and from the pillars of the fornix, but the capsule could not be totally removed.

Follow-up. The postoperative course was complicated by pyogenic meningitis. One month later drainage from the left lateral ventricle was unsatisfactory and Torkildsen's ventriculo-cisternostomy was performed. Recovery was then excellent. Five years later her intellect deteriorated, but radiological investigations did not reveal any obstruction and the ventricular size was unchanged.

Microscopical appearances

The cyst itself is filled with a homogeneous eosinophil core with no cellular constituents. The material stains brightly with periodic acid-Schiff. The wall of the cyst is collagenous, and lined with low cuboidal epithelium. In some places the lining is more complex, formed of layers several cells thick and, here and there, are foci of chronic inflammatory infiltration; within the wall are tubules and clefts lined by the cuboidal epithelium. Cilia and blepharoplasts are not present.

Diagnosis. Colloid cyst.

Summary

The history of sudden falls (drop attacks), preceded by severe headache, is often characteristic of the colloid cyst of the third ventricle. These pedunculated cysts, acting as a ball-valve, may block the foramen of Monro either partially, or completely and acutely.

In this case the cyst was revealed by ventriculogram and then removed. Drainage was required to control the hydrocephalus resulting from obstruction of the ventricle.

Plate 25. COLLOID CYST

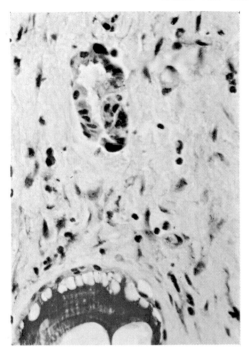

Fig. 1 (Case 21). Edge of the colloid cyst. The contents are Schiff-positive. (PAS × 265)

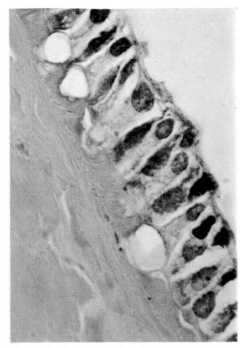

Fig. 2. Another cyst with lining epithelium resembling ependyma. (PTAH × 1060)

PRIMITIVE BIPOTENTIAL TUMOURS;
NEURONAL AND NEURONAL–GLIAL
TUMOURS

MEDULLOBLASTOMA

This is a convenient name for the common malignant tumour of the cerebellum, composed of primitive cells, many of which are probably neuroblastic, while a few are spongioblastic or bipotential. There is evidence that tumours of this type may arise in abnormal proliferation of the fetal granular layer of Obersteiner (Stevenson and Echlin 1934; Kadin et al. 1970), the layer that is responsible for the development of the granule cells of the cerebellum, and that normally disappears soon after birth (*see* Plate 26, Fig. 2). Often subpial spread of the tumour over the surface of the cerebellar folia can mimic the appearance of the Obersteiner layer. Another potential site of origin of medulloblastoma is the neuro-epithelial roof of the fourth ventricle.

The majority of medulloblastomas are found in childhood and early adolescence, but they are not uncommon in the third decade of life and may, rarely, present in the fourth and fifth decades. In childhood the vermis is the usual site, but in adult life the lateral part is more frequently affected and in these cases the presenting symptoms or signs are often not typical of a cerebellar lesion and the course of the disease may be protracted.

The tumours commonly fill the fourth ventricle with growth, and produce hydrocephalus; they frequently metastasize via the cerebrospinal fluid, and leptomeningeal infiltration and dissemination is often extensive (*see* Plate 26, Fig. 4).

The typical microscopical picture is of a highly cellular tumour, rich in small darkly stained nuclei of oval or rounded shape, with little cytoplasm visible. Often the cells are disposed in solid masses, less commonly there are rosettes ('Homer Wright type') or perivascular pseudorosettes; in a number of cases there are microscopical fields that resemble typical oligodendroglioma. Examples are recorded of tumours containing melanin pigment or muscle cells ('medullomyoblastoma'): the latter is regarded as a form of teratoma.

When a medulloblastoma invades the leptomeninges it may stimulate vigorous overgrowth of connective tissue (*see* Plate 28, Fig. 3) and the appearances then produced of islands of tumour cells enclosed in an elaborate reticulin network is known as a 'desmoplastic' medulloblastoma. This is a common mode of growth in the adult (lateral lobe) medulloblastoma and confusion has arisen because some authorities have placed such growths in the category of 'circumscribed arachnoidal sarcoma'. This problem has been discussed in detail by Rubinstein and Northfield (1964).

RETINOBLASTOMA

A highly malignant tumour of the posterior part of the retina presenting similarities to the medulloblastoma: cells with dark-staining close-packed nuclei with little cytoplasm, the frequent formation of Flexner–Wintersteiner rosettes in which cells with peripheral nuclei are grouped around a circular lumen, and extensive propagation via the cerebrospinal fluid with continuous leptomeningeal growth are characteristic.

60

Plate 26. MEDULLOBLASTOMA

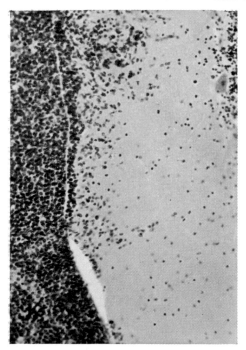

Fig. 1 (Case 22). Medulloblastoma coating the pial surface of the molecular layer of the cerebellum. (H & E   × 105)

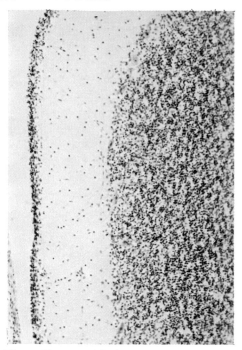

Fig. 2. The normal fetal (external) granular layer of Obersteiner. (Nissl   × 105)

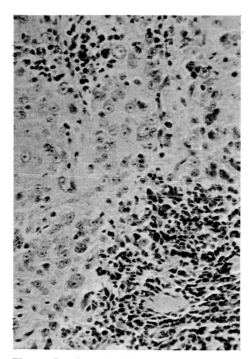

Fig. 3. Ganglion cell differentiation is a notable feature. The small, darkly stained, typical medulloblastoma cells with very little cytoplasm contrast with the much larger ganglion cells with prominent nucleoli and bulky cytoplasm sometimes containing Nissl granules. (H & E   × 210)

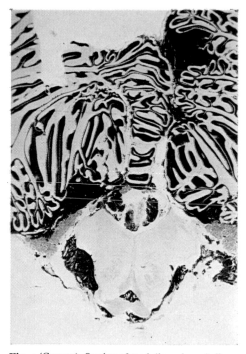

Fig. 4 (Case 22). Section of medulla and cerebellum. Darkly stained masses of tumour coat the meninges in several places and fill the fourth ventricle. (Nissl × 1·6)

Primitive bipotential tumours; neuronal and neuronal-glial tumours

NEUROBLASTOMA; GANGLIOGLIOMA; GANGLIOCYTOMA

Other tumours originating from neuronal or bipotential cells are rare. Cerebral neuro-blastoma is a well-recognized malignant tumour of infancy and childhood whose appearances may be very similar to those of medulloblastoma—small, darkly staining cells with some rosette-formation—or may be more varied. Differentiation into ganglion cells may occur. Invasion of the leptomeninges often results in a marked fibrous tissue reaction (Miller and Ramsden 1966). Gangliocytoma, composed of mature ganglion cells, is very rare in the central nervous system; in the cerebellum a 'dysplastic' variant rarely may be found. Ganglioglioma is a term used for tumours containing both neoplastic ganglionic and glial elements and while usually slow-growing malignant evolution of the glial element can occur. But the diagnosis of ganglioglioma is one that can only be made with considerable caution. Pre-existing neurons are often found intact within astrocytic tumours and in these abnormal conditions may appear atypical. Giant cells in glioblastomas often present bizarre, neuron-like appearances and this should not be taken to indicate neuronal origin. Acceptable cases of gangliocytoma and ganglioglioma have been recorded arising in all parts of the central nervous system; the floor of the third ventricle is the most common. Malignant evolution has been recorded by Russell and Rubinstein (1962). Study of the ultrastructure of ganglioglioma suggests that this tumour may originate from a hamartoma (Rubinstein and Herman 1972).

Bibliography

BAILEY, P. and CUSHING, H. (1925) *Archs Neurol. Psychiat.*, **14**, 192 (Historical).

CHATTY, E. M. and EARLE, K. M. (1971) *Cancer*, **28**, 977 (201 cases).

CHRISTENSEN, E. and ALS, E. (1956) *Acta psychiat. neurol. scand.*, Suppl. 108.

DUCKETT, S. (1963) *Acta psychiat. scand.*, **39**, 242 (Extraneural metastases).

KADIN, M. E., RUBINSTEIN, L. J. and NELSON, J. S. (1970) *J. Neuropath. exp. Neurol.*, **29**, 583 (Origin from fetal granular layer).

KERNOHAN, J. W. and UIHLEIN, A. (1962) *Sarcomas of the Brain*, Chapter 8. Springfield, Ill.: Charles C Thomas (Discussion of cerebellar arachnoidal sarcoma).

PATERSON, E. (1961) *Brain*, **84**, 301 (Extradural metastases).

POLAK, M. (1967) *Acta neuropath.*, **8**, 84 (Neuroblastic nature).

RUBINSTEIN, L. J. (1972) *J. Neuropath. exp. Neurol.*, **31**, 7 (Review of histogenesis of medulloblastoma and other primitive tumours).

RUBINSTEIN, L. J. and NORTHFIELD, D. W. C. (1964) *Brain*, **87**, 379 (Medulloblastoma and cerebellar arachnoidal sarcoma).

SPITZ, E. B., SHENKIN, H. A. and GRANT, F. C. (1947) *Archs Neurol. Psychiat.*, **57**, 417 (Cases in adults: different survival periods).

STEVENSON, L. and ECHLIN, F. (1934) *Archs Neurol. Psychiat.*, **31**, 93 (Origin from fetal granular layer).

Neuroblastoma (cerebral)

MILLER, A. A. and RAMSDEN, F. (1966) *J. Neuropath. exp. Neurol.*, **25**, 328 (Desmoplastic reaction).

Ganglioglioma

RUBINSTEIN, L. J. and HERMAN, M. M. (1972) *J. neurol. Sci.*, **16**, 27.

RUSSELL, DOROTHY S. and RUBINSTEIN, L. J. (1962) *J. Neuropath. exp. Neurol.*, **21**, 185.

MEDULLOBLASTOMA

Case 22. Male infant 2½ years

History. Six weeks' left sided ptosis of sudden onset. Admitted to hospital and found to have left third and seventh nerve palsies. No cause could be found. Cerebrospinal fluid protein 56 mg/100 ml. Discharged from hospital. Two weeks' occipital headaches, vomiting and unsteady gait led to readmission.

Examination. Bilateral papilloedema. Complete left third cranial nerve palsy and seventh nerve palsy. Walking on a very broad base, tending to fall backwards.

Progress. Cardiac and respiratory arrest before any investigation or treatment could be started.

Necropsy. Soft, pink-grey, homogeneous tumour was infiltrating both cerebellar hemispheres, filling the aqueduct, fourth and third ventricles, and spreading in the leptomeninges from the optic tract to the spinal cord. The lateral ventricles were dilated. There was no extraneural tumour.

Microscopical appearances

The tumour forms several solid masses within the cerebellar hemispheres and extends in the leptomeninges, covering the folia with thick sheets of growth which here and there penetrate the molecular layer. The cells are small, with round or oval vesicular nuclei and little stainable cytoplasm and are very similar to, but slightly larger than, the granule cells of the cerebellum. There are no glial fibres. Rosette formation is sparse. Collagen and reticulin are restricted to blood vessels. In the leptomeninges over the cord there is extension of the tumour with a few strands of reticulin between cells.

Diagnosis. Medulloblastoma.

Summary

This child died suddenly before any investigations were made. Patients with posterior fossa tumours of all types are particularly liable to die unexpectedly from acute medullary compression.

Extensive spread of the cerebellar neoplasm was found from the optic chiasm to the lumbar spinal cord. Medulloblastoma is a highly cellular, malignant tumour with a tendency to behave as though it had been poured widely over the leptomeninges in a fluid state: for this reason radiotherapy is given to the whole neuraxis.

Plate 27. MEDULLOBLASTOMA

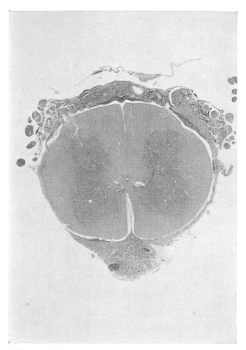

Fig. 1 (Case 22). Spinal cord ensheathed with medulloblastoma. (H & E   × 5·5)

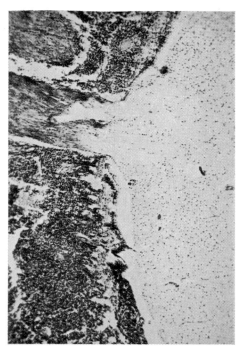

Fig. 2 (Case 22). Darkly stained masses of tumour extend in the leptomeninges on either side of a posterior nerve root entering the cord. (Nissl × 45)

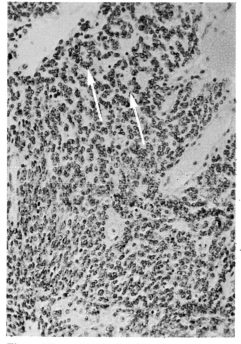

Fig. 3. The typical medulloblastoma appearances: cells with small darkly stained nuclei and negligible cytoplasm sometimes arranged in small rosettes (arrows). (H & E   × 175)

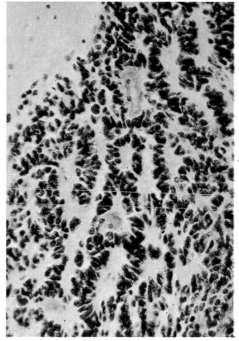

Fig. 4. In this example there is conspicuous peri-vascular 'pseudorosette' formation. (H van Gieson × 210)

MEDULLOBLASTOMA
Case 23. Man aged 51

History. Three months' bifrontal headache, followed by severe throbbing left frontal headache extending behind the left eye. One week's severe stabbing pain over the vertex radiating to the back of the neck, vomiting and unsteadiness.

Examination. Mentally normal. Slight weakness of left arm and cerebellar incoordination of left side of body.

Investigations. Lumbar puncture revealed xanthochromic fluid. Carotid and vertebral angiograms normal. Air encephalogram: no air entered ventricles but the brain-stem and basal cisterns appeared normal.

Clinical diagnosis. Subarachnoid haemorrhage. Aneurysm?

Follow-up. He was now free of headache and was discharged with no abnormality on physical examination. Two months later he developed nausea and vomiting and was readmitted. He was mentally retarded and there were signs of left hemiparesis involving arm and leg, left-sided cerebellar incoordination and ataxic gait. Blood pressure was 90/60. Repeated angiograms were unhelpful. He died without diagnosis.

Necropsy. A soft, creamy and pink coloured partly necrotic tumour 4 cm in diameter occupied much of the left cerebellar hemisphere. It infiltrated the leptomeninges and was adherent to the dura. Death was attributed to medullary compression. No extracranial tumour was found.

Microscopical appearances

The tumour is very cellular and in some places necrotic. The cells have oval or round darkly stained nuclei and sparse cytoplasm; rarely they resemble the cells of an oligodendroglioma with larger, round nuclei with a clear perinuclear 'halo'. There are cellular rosettes and perivascular pseudo-rosettes. Connective tissue is varied in amount; especially where the growth has invaded the meninges the amount of reticulin fibres is large and here the tumour cells are clustered in groups ('pale islands') separated by bands of fibres. Another pattern is formed by the connective tissue separating the tumour into short narrow rows and sinuous trabeculae.

Diagnosis. Medulloblastoma corresponding to the 'desmoplastic' type described by Rubinstein and Northfield.

Summary

The original clinical diagnosis of subarachnoid haemorrhage due to an aneurysm was not confirmed by the arteriograms. Following the air study the patient appeared perfectly well and no further investigations were undertaken. On his second admission extensive investigations were made, but no diagnosis was indicated.

Medulloblastoma is a recognized tumour in adults, though considerably less common than in children and in adolescents. It tends to involve the lateral parts rather than the vermis, and the presenting symptoms may not be typical of a cerebellar tumour. The tempo of the disease is often slower, but extensive leptomeningeal spread will eventually occur.

Plate 28. MEDULLOBLASTOMA

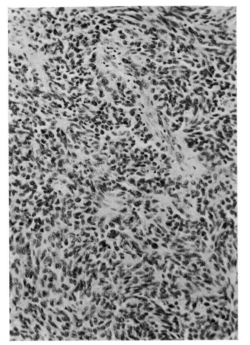

Fig. 1 (Case 23). A low power view showing the dense cellularity of the tumour. (Nissl × 105)

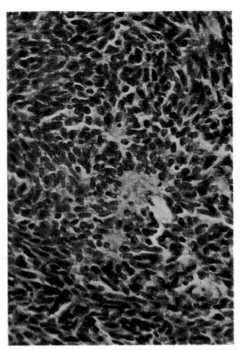

Fig. 2 (Case 23). Cells with dark-staining oval nuclei in a densely packed mass. Some rosettes are present. (Nissl × 265)

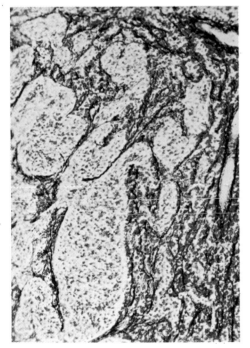

Fig. 3. In parts of the tumour reticulin fibrils are numerous. In other places clear islands of cells are enclosed by the fibrils. (Reticulin × 105)

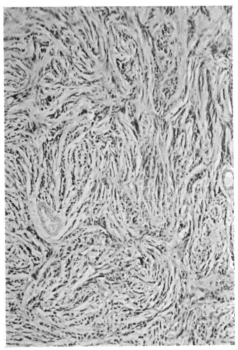

Fig. 4 (Case 23). Sinuous linear trabeculae of medulloblastoma cells. (H & E × 105)

Tumours of lymphoreticular cells

Synonyms: microglioma; reticulum cell sarcoma; malignant lymphoma of brain; reticulo-histiocytic encephalitis etc.

Tumours of lymphoreticular cells are less common than astrocytomas or glioblastomas.

Despite the semantic confusion indicated by the many synonyms the pathological findings do not show much variation from case to case. There may be diffuse infiltration, apparent to the naked eye as swelling or blurring of normal structures, or a well-defined mass of pale grey, sometimes necrotic, tumour. Microscopical examination usually reveals unexpectedly extensive infiltration. The cells distend the perivascular spaces and infiltrate the nearby neural tissue to form a tumour of any size from a minute solitary focus to a large confluent mass. The leptomeninges are often involved. The cellular morphology varies: many cells have irregular chromatin networks, often multiple nucleoli, and sparse eosinophil cytoplasm (*see* Plate 29, Fig. 1); less common are multinucleate giant cells. The mitotic incidence is generally high. More mature cells resemble microglia and are often metallophil when suitable silver impregnation methods are applied. Some tumour cells may be phagocytic (*see* Plate 29, Fig. 2). In rare cases plasma cells are numerous. At the margins of the infiltration perivascular lymphocytic cuffing, and a marked astrocytic reaction, are usual (*see* Plate 29, Fig. 3). Reticulin methods reveal a characteristic lamellar pattern of split fibrils within a distended perivascular space (*see* Plate 29, Fig. 4).

In a number of cases (less than a half of those recorded) the nervous system lesions are accompanied by lymphoma in extraneural sites. There is an interesting, but at present unexplained, association between these tumours and disorders of immunity (such as the Wiskott–Aldrich syndrome), and organ transplant patients on immunosuppressive therapy carry a specially high risk (Hoover and Fraumeni 1973).

When systemic lymphomas such as Hodgkin's disease or lymphosarcoma involve the nervous system a different pattern is usually presented. The infiltration frequently affects the meninges and nerve roots, rarely the parenchyma, and is commoner in the spine than in the cranium. The optic nerves may be involved. Spinal cord compression resulting from epidural masses is one common type of presentation and peripheral neuropathy may result from extensive permeation of the nerve bundles by malignant cells.

In the leukaemias widespread leptomeningeal infiltration is a frequent complication, present in the majority of cases in childhood.

Bibliography

ADAMS, J. H. and JACKSON, J. M. (1966) *J. Path. Bact.*, **91**, 369 (Pathology of microglioma).
FRENCH, J. D. (1947) *J. Neuropath. exp. Neurol.*, **6**, 265.
HOOVER, R. and FRAUMENI, J. F., jun. (1973) *Lancet*, **2**, 55
JELLINGER, K. and SEITELBERGER, F. (1975) *Acta neuropath.*, Suppl. VI. (Includes several valuable papers).
RUSSELL, DOROTHY S., MARSHALL, A. H. E. and SMITH, F. B. (1948) *Brain*, **71**, 1 (Microglioma).
SCHAUMBURG, H. H., PLANK, C. R. and ADAMS, R. D. (1972) *Brain*, **95**, 199.
WILLIAMS, H. M., DIAMOND, H. D., CRAVER, L. F. and PARSONS, H. (1959) *Neurological Complications of Lymphomas and Leukaemias*. Springfield, Ill.; Charles C Thomas.

Plate 29. LYMPHORETICULAR TUMOUR

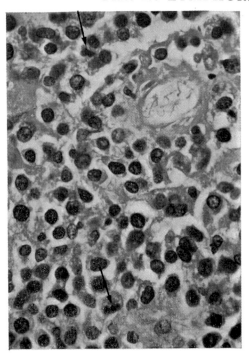

Fig. 1 (Case 24). Lymphoreticular cells clustered in a Virchow-Robin space. The cells have vesicular nuclei, often with prominent nucleoli, and an indistinct rim of eosinophil cytoplasm. (H & E   × 420)

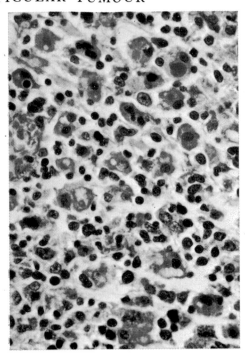

Fig. 2. Mixed cell population in a microglioma. Some large phagocytic cells contain Schiff-positive material in their cytoplasm. (PAS   × 265)

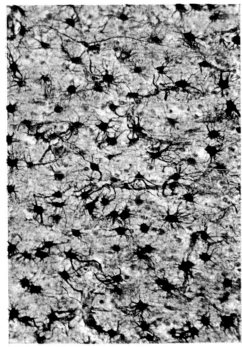

Fig. 3 (Case 24). Numerous large fibrous astrocytes near the periphery of the tumorous infiltration. (Cajal's gold sublimate   × 265)

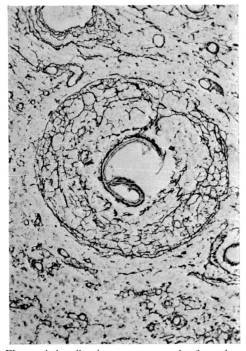

Fig. 4. A lamellated appearance results from the splitting and fragmentation of the periadventitial reticulin fibres of a small vessel. (Reticulin × 105)

LYMPHORETICULAR TUMOUR

Case 24. Man aged 51

History. Ten days' loss of concentration and breathlessness with hyperventilation. He was found to have marked respiratory alkalosis and hypokalaemia due to persistent hyperventilation of central origin. After two weeks signs suggesting a left hemisphere lesion appeared.

Examination. Persistent overbreathing (rate 36/min). Conscious, with poor memory and concentration. Dyspraxic. Eyes deviated to right but no loss of conjugate gaze. Bilateral grasp reflex. Right hemiparesis, predominantly in leg. Possible sensory loss on right side of body.

Clinical diagnosis. Neurogenic hyperventilation (cause ?). Left hemisphere tumour (nature ?).

Investigations. Left carotid angiogram indicated a temporal mass extending deeply.

Operation. Anterior temporal, posterior parietal and occipital burrhole biopsies. The intracranial pressure was greatly raised. No mass could be felt on needling; portions of softened brain were aspirated.

Follow-up. Conscious state fluctuated; hyperventilation continued. Died ten days later.

Necropsy. Diffuse pale grey tumour in left temporo-occipital white matter with great oedema. Diffuse enlargement (from infiltration) of upper pons. Small nodules (up to 1 cm in diameter) of tumour in liver.

Microscopical appearances

Aspiration biopsies. Grey and white matter infiltrated with perivascular clusters of neoplastic cells. Tumour of reticular tissue suggested.

Post-mortem. The tumour spreads diffusely through the white matter. The leptomeninges are heavily infiltrated and thick cuffs of cells extend into the cortex along the perivascular spaces. Many of the cells are immature lymphoreticular cells with oval vesicular nuclei, prominent nucleoli and hazy, ill-defined cytoplasm of no regular shape. Amongst these primitive cells there are other smaller cells with bilobed nuclei that resemble microglia as well as some cells with eccentric 'spotty' nuclei resembling plasma cell precursors. Mitotic figures are fairly numerous. Silver impregnations reveal metallophilia of many of the tumour cells and demonstrate numbers of mature microglia. Between the groups of neoplastic cells and around the margins of the deposits, there are numerous large fibre-forming astrocytes. The reticulin of the walls of the infiltrated vessels is split into concentric laminae by the proliferating cells. In the brain-stem the diffuse infiltration involves mainly the mid-brain and fibre-bundles of the upper pons. There are foci of infiltration in other parts of the brain only visible on microscopical examination. The tumours in the liver are malignant lymphoma.

Diagnosis. Primary tumour of lymphoreticular cells ('microglioma').

Summary

An extensive, multifocal tumour involving the brain and upper brain-stem, presenting with signs of neurogenic hyperventilation and left hemisphere mass. The pathological findings are typical of microglioma.

Plate 30. LYMPHORETICULAR TUMOUR

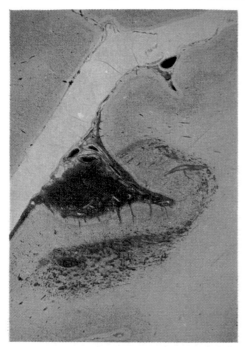

Fig. 1 (Case 24). At low power, heavy leptomeningeal infiltration and perivascular penetration of the cortex and infiltration of the white matter are evident. This focus is separate from the main tumour mass (Celloidin) (Nissl × 3·2)

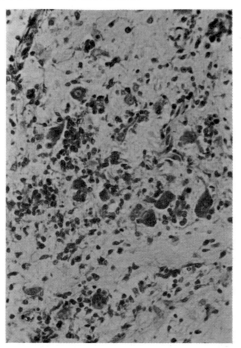

Fig. 2 (Case 24). Infiltration of the upper pons. The cells are spreading from the affected perivascular spaces to cluster around pontine neurons. (Celloidin) (Nissl × 210)

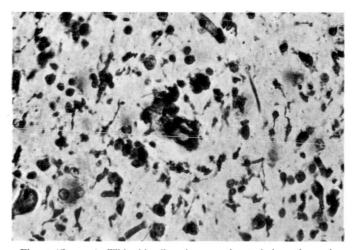

Fig. 3 (Case 24). With this silver impregnation technique the perivascular tumour cells are darkly stained and numerous active microglia (mainly in the elongated form) are revealed. (Frozen section) (Naoumenko–Feigin × 265)

SYSTEMIC LYMPHOMA—HODGKIN'S DISEASE

Case 25. Woman aged 25

History. (Past) One year previously, investigation of chest symptoms revealed a large tumour in left side of chest adherent to lung and diaphragm. Histology inconclusive. Remained with pyrexia, high sedimentation rate, anaemia and hepatomegaly. (Present) Six months' difficulty in walking, 'stocking' paraesthesiae in both legs, with 'burning' of feet; three months' urgency of micturition; two weeks' pain in midthoracic region of spine radiating around chest and progressive weakness of legs. 'Burning' of legs replaced by numbness. Headache mainly at the back of the head, present on waking. Double vision on looking to the right. Three days' total leg paralysis.

Examination. Pale, cachectic, febrile. Liver enlarged. Tenderness over the spine at D6–7 Neck stiffness. Right sixth cranial nerve palsy. Wasting of the right side of the tongue. Paraplegia with motor and sensory levels at D6: no voluntary movement of lower limbs.

Investigations. Haemoglobin 10·4 g/100 ml. ESR 90 mm/hour (Westergren). Leucocytes 13 000/mm³ (neutrophils 92 per cent). Radiograph of skull and whole length of spine, no abnormality. Lumbar myelogram showed block at D8. CSF (lumbar): protein 400 mg/ml, no cells. Cisternal myelogram: complete obstruction to flow at D6. CSF (cisternal): protein 42 mg/100 ml, 4 lymphocytes. Appearances suggested an extradural mass compressing the theca.

Operation. Laminectomy D6, 7, 8, 9. A plaque of hard grey tumour presented on the posterior aspect of the theca embracing it on both sides. All obvious neoplasm was removed.

Follow-up. Postoperatively some sensation returned to both legs, but no movement. Three months later she died after developing *grand mal* epilepsy. At necropsy a large mass of tumour filled the mediastinum and infiltrated both lungs. The para-aortic lymph nodes were enlarged, whence the growth had spread to the adjacent vertebrae and involved the spinal canal from D6 to L1. There were large tumour masses in the meninges over the left frontal lobe and medulla.

Microscopical appearances

Much of the tumour tissue received is necrotic. The viable tissue is composed of a mixture of cell types including lymphocytes, fibroblasts and leucocytes and a relatively large number of atypical reticulum cells with large single or double nuclei containing prominent nucleoli (Sternberg–Reed cells).

Diagnosis. Hodgkin's disease.

Summary

The original biopsy of the intrathoracic tumour revealed fibrotic tissue: sclerosis is the usual sequel to granulomatous Hodgkin's disease.

Signs of cord compression may be a presenting feature of Hodgkin's disease in the central nervous system. Epilepsy, resulting from meningeal deposits, which may mimic a meningioma, is a less frequent symptom. In only a very small number of cases of this lymphoma has infiltration of the brain substance been reported.

Other forms of neural involvement, especially in treated cases, include a variety of opportunistic infections, progressive multifocal leucoencephalopathy and post-irradiation necrosis.

Plate 31. SYSTEMIC LYMPHOMA—HOGDKIN'S DISEASE

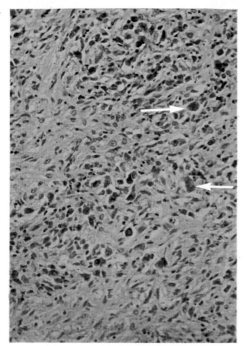

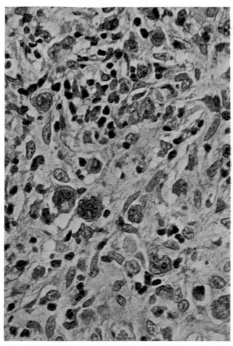

Fig. 1 (Case 25). Atypical reticulum cells including giant cells (arrows), fibroblasts, lymphocytes and macrophages. (H & E   × 175)

Fig. 2 (Case 25). Atypical reticulum cells with multiple nuclei (Sternberg–Reed cells), fibroblasts, lymphocytes and macrophages. (H & E   × 420)

MYELOMA
Case 26. Man aged 43

History. Eight months' pain in the right side of the neck and right arm, with radiation to the right wrist, chiefly in the evening. One month previously he felt a 'click' in the neck on turning the head. Pain exacerbated ever since.

Examination. Mentally normal. Tenderness over spine C7–D1. Marked restriction of all movements of neck by pain; wasting and weakness of right deltoid, triceps and interossei with hypotonia and reduced reflexes. Tone increased and limb reflexes exaggerated in both lower limbs.

Investigations. Radiographs of the spine revealed destruction of the right side of the bodies, transverse processes, pedicles and laminae of C6, C7 and D1. Myelogram showed a block at the level of the bony lesions with cord displacement to left, suggesting extradural mass on right. Haemoglobin 12·7 g/100 ml. ESR 91 mm/hour (Westergren). Leucocytes 14000/mm³. Blood film: many of the lymphoid cells large, resembling immature plasma cells. Protein strip revealed an abnormal band close to the gamma position.

Clinical differential diagnosis. Myeloma or other lymphoma? Secondary carcinoma? Aneurysmal bone cyst?

Operation. Cervical laminectomy. Tumour tissue was present in the paraspinal muscles, and at C7 and D1 the entire lamina was replaced by tumour and there were no pedicles remaining. As much as possible of the tumour was removed and the C8 and D1 nerve roots on the right side, which were involved in the growth, were cleared. No attempt was made at anterior removal because of the danger from haemorrhage.

Follow-up. After a course of radiotherapy and chemotherapy he was able to return to work wearing a special collar. Two months later the pain in the neck had diminished. Eighteen months later he had discarded the collar and reported that he was able to lead a fairly normal life.

Microscopical appearances

The tumour is intensely cellular and is composed of mononuclear cells of varied outline, possessing differing amounts of eosinophil cytoplasm and oval vesicular nuclei. The nuclear chromatin is characteristically 'spotty'. The most mature cells are typical plasma cells with eccentric 'clockface' nuclei. Unna–Pappenheim's method demonstrates marked affinity for pyronin.

Diagnosis. Myeloma (plasmacytoma).

Summary

In this case cord compression was associated with destructive lesions in the spine and an extra-dural mass. Laboratory investigations strongly suggested myeloma, and this diagnosis was confirmed. The operation was successful, and while manifestations of multiple bony lesions must be considered a likely future development, no signs have appeared so far.

Myeloma often involves the skull, and while the dura may be infiltrated, penetration of the brain is extremely rare.

A single case of a plasma-celled tumour involving the third ventricle was recorded by French (1947).

Plate 32. MYELOMA

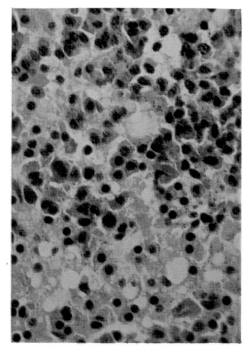

Fig. 1 (Case 26). Many of the cells resemble mature plasma cells with 'spotty' nuclear chromatin; others are larger and less typical. (H & E   × 530)

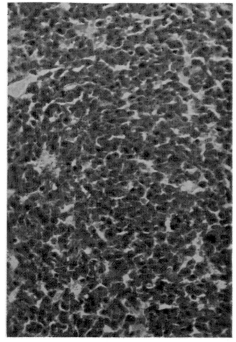

Fig. 2 (Case 26). Intense pyronin staining of cells. (Unna–Pappenheim (methyl green pyronin)   × 210)

Blood-vessel tumours and malformations

TUMOURS

The capillary haemangioblastoma (haemangio-endothelioma) is a well-localized benign tumour that may be found in the cerebellum (usually as a nodule within a cyst), in the pia covering the medulla or spinal cord, or within the orbit. It comprises a network of capillary-size and larger blood vessels, lined by endothelial cells, with intervening stromal cells which often contain much foamy lipid material (Plate 33, Fig. 2). Abnormally high levels of haemoglobin have been recorded in some cases, due to erythropoietically-active substances in the cyst fluid.

These growths may be single or multiple. Familial cases associated with extraneural lesions such as cysts in the pancreas and kidney, renal carcinoma, and phaeochromocytoma are known as Lindau's disease; in the von Hippel variant there is coexisting retinal haemangioblastoma.

MALFORMATIONS

The *capillary angioma* (telangiectasis) consists of capillary size, thin-walled vessels, lined with a single endothelial layer and clustered in lobules or distributed diffusely. It is most common in the brain-stem. The *cavernous angioma*, most frequently found in the cortex or subcortical white matter, has very large vessels whose walls contain varied amounts of connective tissue (*see* Plate 36, Fig. 2) and which sometimes contain thrombus. No normal neural tissue separates these distended vessels, which are often calcified.

There is no sharp demarcation between these two types and there may be transitions.

In Sturge-Weber's disease an extensive vascular malformation of one cerebral hemisphere is associated with a 'port-wine stain' facial naevus on the same side. A distinctive feature is the presence of cortical calcification with a 'tramline' radiographic pattern (Plate 33, Fig. 1).

In *arteriovenous malformations*, which vary considerably in size, some being very extensive, abnormal arterial and venous channels communicate. Microscopically the vessels are quite abnormal and it may be difficult to decide whether they are truly arterial or venous. Hyaline thickening of the vessels, thrombosis and calcification are usual.

Bibliography

AMINOFF, M. J. and LOGUE, V. (1974) *Brain*, **97**, 211.
CRAMER, F. and KINSEY, W. (1952) *Archs Neurol. Psychiat.*, **67**, 237.
PATERSON, J. H. and MCKISSOCK, W. (1956) *Brain*, **79**, 233 (110 cases of intracranial angiomas, discussion of natural history and treatment).
SARGENT, P. and GREENFIELD, J. G. (1929) *Br. J. Surg.*, **17**, 84 (Haemangioblastoma cerebelli).
WEBER, F. P. (1929) *Proc. R. Soc. Med.*, **22**, 431 (Association of facial naevus with calcified cerebral angioma).
WYBURN-MASON, R. (1943) *The Vascular Abnormalities and Tumours of the Spinal Cord and its Membranes*. London: Kimpton.

Plate 33. BLOOD-VESSEL TUMOURS

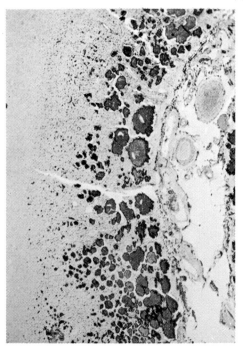

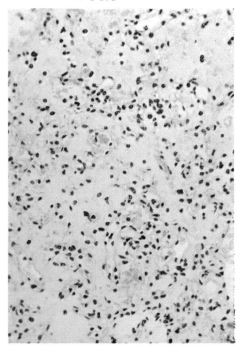

Fig. 1. Sturge-Weber's disease. Abnormal, angio-matous vessels are present in the meninges. There is abundant calcification of the outer laminae of the cortex. (H & E   × 26)

Fig. 2. Haemangioblastoma in the pia mater of the spinal cord. These tumours are similar to the com-moner cerebellar examples. (H & E   × 420)

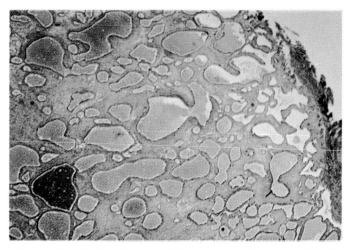

Fig. 3. An orbital angioma consisting of a mass of large blood-filled spaces in a connective-tissue network. (Reticulin   × 26)

HAEMANGIOBLASTOMA

Case 27. Woman aged 20

History. (Past) Right eye blind for eight years; enucleated three years previously (retinal haemangioblastoma). (Present) Two months' pain in back of the head without nausea, daily. Two weeks' sudden blurring of vision on standing up, occurring about six times.

Examination. Papilloedema with haemorrhages and exudates. Left sixth nerve paresis. Left lower motor neuron facial weakness.

Clinical diagnosis. Haemangioblastoma cerebelli most likely even in the absence of cerebellar disturbance.

Investigations. Haemoglobin 13·2 g/100 ml. Left carotid angiogram showed no ventricular enlargement. Left vertebral angiogram indicated the presence of two haemangioblastoma nodules in the left cerebellar hemisphere supplied by the posterior inferior cerebellar artery.

Operation. Posterior fossa craniotomy. A cyst containing 25 ml of clear yellow fluid was found in the left cerebellar hemisphere and aspirated. The two cherry-red tumour nodules in the cerebellum were joined by an isthmus: the lateral one presented onto the surface, the medial one into the cyst. Numerous blood vessels derived from both superficial and deep vessels ran into each tumour. They were removed completely; the larger was 2 × 1 cm, the smaller 1·2 cm in diameter. A third small red nodule was found on the surface of the right cerebellar hemisphere and excised.

Follow-up. Five years later well with no recurrence.

Microscopical appearances

A rim of haemorrhagic cerebellar folia surrounds a circumscribed nodule composed of an elaborate network of small and moderate sized blood spaces lined with cells of epithelial type. The capillary pattern of this network is best seen in the sections impregnated for reticulin. The stroma contains a few polygonal cells with foamy cytoplasm and central spheroidal nuclei. Review of the section of the eye earlier removed revealed a tumour of similar type.

Diagnosis. Capillary haemangioblastoma. Von Hippel–Lindau's syndrome.

Summary

The possibility of a cerebellar tumour in this case was first raised by the past history, and was favoured despite normal tests of cerebellar function. The appearance of a cyst filled with yellow liquid and containing a red mural nodule is diagnostic.

The presence of multiple cerebellar nodules is characteristic of the familial cases (von Hippel–Lindau).

Plate 34. HAEMANGIOBLASTOMA

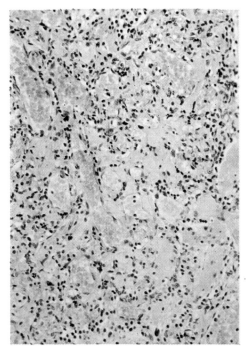

Fig. 1 (Case 27). A meshwork of blood-filled spaces enclosed in a cellular framework. (H van Gieson × 130)

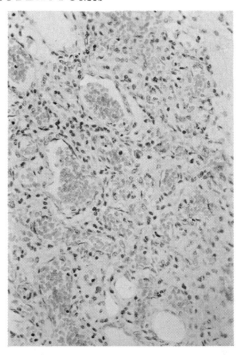

Fig. 2. Some larger blood-filled spaces amongst the capillaries. (H & E × 130)

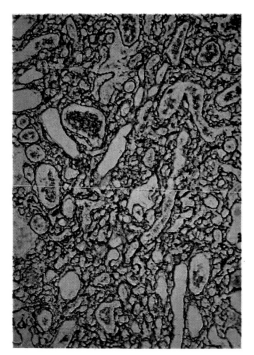

Fig. 3 (Case 27). Reticulin impregnation outlines the structure of the capillary network. (Reticulin × 105)

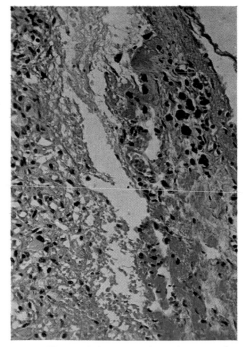

Fig. 4. Pigment-laden macrophages in connective tissue at the margin of tumour. (H van Gieson × 210)

CAVERNOUS ANGIOMA

Case 28. Man aged 41

History. Two years' intermittent back pain while lying down. Nine months' difficulty in walking on a straight line and weakness in legs below the knees. Three months' numbness in left leg.

Examination. Wasting of right thigh and calf muscles. Weakness of right hip flexors and of dorsiflexors of ankles and toes. Reduction of all modalities of sensation on the left over the L2–5 segments. Loss of vibration sense on both sides up to iliac crest. Bilateral extensor plantar responses.

Investigations. Radiographs of the dorsal spine showed erosion of the right D9 pedicle. Myelogram showed almost complete obstruction at the level of D10. The theca was displaced towards the left by a mass on its right lateral aspect.

Operation. Laminectomy D8, 9, 10. Encapsulated very vascular purple tumour protruded as soon as the D10 lamina was removed. It measured 4 × 3 × 1·5 cm and had displaced the dura far over to the left. It was dissected out completely after a leash of arteries entering the tumour from the intervertebral foramen had been divided.

Follow-up. At discharge, slight right-sided weakness but no sensory deficit. Eighteen months later he was well.

Microscopical appearances

The tumour is formed by a network of blood-filled spaces, varying in size from capillaries to large sinusoids, separated by stromal connective tissue containing flattened endothelial and fibroblastic cells. No mitoses are seen. The stromal elements do not resemble meningeal cells.

Diagnosis. Cavernous angioma.

Summary

The cavernous angioma is a vascular malformation most commonly found in the cerebrum. In this case it presented as an extradural tumour producing signs of compression of the spinal cord in the lower thoracic region, a less common situation. It was completely removed.

Microscopically there was a mixture of large vascular spaces with hyaline walls and smaller ones resembling dilated capillaries.

Plate 35. CAVERNOUS ANGIOMA

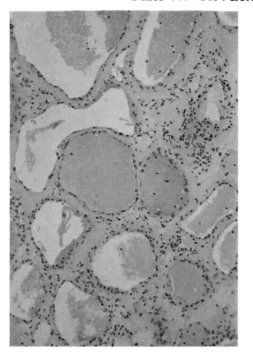

Fig. 1 (Case 28). Rounded blood-filled spaces lined by a single endothelial layer. (H & E × 105)

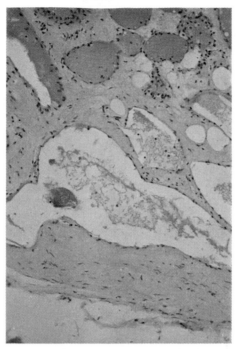

Fig. 2 (Case 28). Vascular channels of varied size lying in a connective tissue stroma. (H & E × 105)

CAVERNOUS ANGIOMA

Case 29. Woman aged 23

History. (Past) Age 7 to 20: episodes of frontal headache, nausea and vomiting, lasting one day and occurring about once a month—diagnosed as migraine. Age 20: schizophrenia diagnosed—treated with ECT. Age 22: occasional episodes of 'automatic behaviour' in which she became mute and inaccessible. (Present) Two days' headache and nausea; found unconscious.

Examination. Drowsy, confused, disorientated in time and space, perseverating. Neck stiffness, Kernig's sign present. Right hemiparesis (mild). Restriction of all voluntary eye movements especially on upward and lateral gaze.

Investigations. Lumbar puncture: heavily blood-stained CSF with yellow supernatant. Bilateral carotid angiograms revealed an angioma about 1 cm in diameter in the left temporal lobe supplied by a greatly enlarged left anterior choroidal artery.

Operation. Left temporal craniotomy. The surface of the brain was normal. In the floor of the temporal horn a large vein emerging from the angioma was found. Blood clot occupying the temporal horn was sucked away. The large anterior choroidal artery was clipped and divided and the anterior part of the lobe bearing the angioma on its deep surface lifted out.

Follow-up. Immediate postoperative dysphasia and dyslexia, which improved progressively.

Microscopical appearances

The cortex is fenestrated by a plexus of abnormal blood vessels of irregular shape whose walls are of very variable thickness and have no proper structure, being composed of collagenous connective tissue with a few disarranged elastic fibres, and with occasional focal calcification. There are also a few arteries of normal appearance. Tongues of gliotic tissue surround some of the vessels.

Diagnosis. Cavernous angioma.

Summary

The long history of episodic headache, vomiting and psychological disturbances suggested a slowly progressive temporal lobe lesion. The illness culminated in an acute haemorrhage.

The cortical cavernous angiomas are often associated with focal epilepsy; those involving the third and fourth ventricles may produce hydrocephalus. As with other hamartomas they often form a part of a picture of multiple developmental errors: angiomas and telangiectasis in the nervous system (possibly affecting several sites) can be accompanied by similar lesions or by cysts elsewhere in the body.

Plate 36. CAVERNOUS ANGIOMA

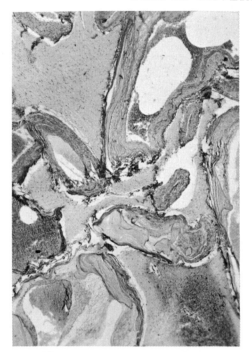

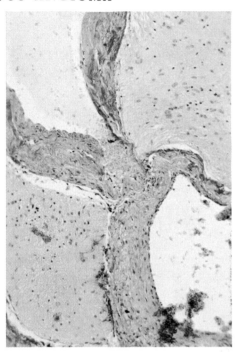

Fig. 1 (Case 29). A group of abnormal blood vessels. Some resemble arteries, with prominent elastic coats, in others the walls are simply connective tissue of varied thickness. (H van Gieson   × 105)

Fig. 2. Detail of cavernous blood channel. There is a single endothelial lining and a collagenous wall. (H van Gieson   × 265)

ANGIOMA OF SPINAL CORD

Case 30. Man aged 38

History. Two years' progressive weakness and clumsiness of right leg.

Examination. Impairment of all modalities of sensation below D8; spastic paresis.

Investigations. Myelogram indicated extensive tortuous vessels typical of an angioma.

Follow-up. The patient developed total paraplegia with loss of all modalities of sensation below the level of the umbilicus. He died eight years later.

Necropsy. Extensive angioma of the cord, consisting of dilated vessels forming a tortuous plexus in the leptomeninges. The largest feeding vessel to penetrate the dura ran with the posterior root of D8. At this level, and below, the cord was stained dark brown and softened.

Microscopical appearances

In the leptomeninges there are several very large abnormal blood vessels mainly of arterial type. There is extensive infarction of the cord at the centre of which is a cystic cavity. All around this zone of softening there are innumerable tiny blood vessels whose walls are hyaline connective tissue.

Diagnosis. Angioma of spinal cord.

Summary

Spinal angiomas (known as Foix-Alajouanine disease) consist of anomalous vessels with arterio-venous communications in the leptomeninges and within the cord substance. They may present with acute symptoms, due to haemorrhage, or with subacute symptoms which may be exacerbated by exercise, certain postures or pregnancy. The diagnosis is made by myelography and confirmed by selective spinal angiography. In the case described the patient died with paraplegia due to infarction of the cord eight years after the diagnosis had been made. Today such patients can be treated successfully by excision of the malformation.

Plate 37. ANGIOMA OF SPINAL CORD

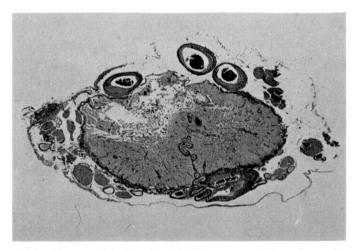

Fig. 1 (Case 30). Spinal cord at D8. There are several large abnormal blood vessels in the leptomeninges. The large cystic cavity is the result of infarction. (H van Gieson   × 4·5)

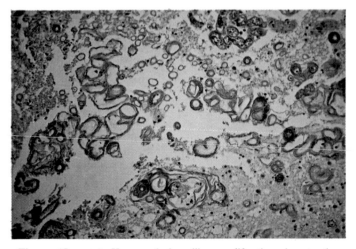

Fig. 2. (Case 30). Very marked capillary proliferation close to the infarction. (H van Gieson   × 105)

Pituitary and parapituitary tumours

ADENOMA

Adenomas of the anterior pituitary have been classified according to the cell types (Plate 38, Fig. 4) into chromophobe (79 per cent), acidophil (15 per cent) and basophil (6 per cent) (Russell and Rubinstein 1971). A proportion are of mixed type.

Chromophobe adenomas often attain large size, expand the sella turcica, compress the optic chiasm, displace the third ventricle and may infiltrate the cavernous sinuses. Acidophil and basophil adenomas are usually smaller and restricted to within the sella; their presence is more often revealed by symptoms of endocrine imbalance than by those of space-occupation. Although chromophobe and mixed adenomas may display invasive behaviour it is rare for them to exhibit true malignancy, as judged either by the production of metastases or by variation in the histological appearances.

Tumours of the neurohypophysis ('pituicytoma', 'granular cell myoblastoma') are rare.

CRANIOPHARYNGIOMA

This is the most convenient name for the solid and cystic suprasellar tumours believed to be derived from Rathke's pouch. Synonyms include 'adamantinoma' and 'suprasellar epidermoid'. While many examples of these lesions are discovered in childhood, others present in adult life. The cystic examples carry a better prognosis than the solid. In appearance they are often shiny and semi-translucent, enclosed within a distinct capsule, and sometimes contain solid calcified particles. Cholesterol crystals may be found in the cyst fluid. Escape of the contents may provoke meningitis.

Microscopical appearances are of cystic or solid masses of epithelial tumour (*see* Plate 42, Figs 1–3). The cells may be columnar, lining numerous cystic spaces, or squamous and associated with quantities of lamellated keratin which may undergo calcification. Malignant changes do not occur.

Bibliography

Adenomas
CUSHING, H. (1912) *The Pituitary Body and Its Disorders*. Philadelphia: Lippincott.
CUSHING, H. (1932) *Johns Hopkins Hosp. Bull.*, **50**, 137 (Basophil adenoma).
JEFFERSON, G. (1955) *The Invasive Adenomas of the Anterior Pituitary*. Liverpool: Liverpool University Press.
KERNOHAN, J. W. and SAYRE, G. P. (1956) *Tumors of Pituitary Gland and Infundibulum. Atlas of Tumor Pathology*, Fascicle 26. Washington, D.C.: Armed Forces Institute of Pathology.
RAY, B. S. and other authors (1962) *J. Neurosurg.*, **19**, 1 (Symposium on pituitary tumours).
ROVIT, R. L. and BERRY, R. (1965) *J. Neurosurg.*, **23**, 270 (Discussion of hyperadrenalism and pituitary tumours).
RUSSELL, DOROTHY S. and RUBINSTEIN, L. J. (1971) See p. x.

Craniopharyngiomas
BARTLETT, J. R. (1971) *J. Neurol. Neurosurg. Psychiat.*, **34**, 37 (Summary of eighty-five cases).
NORTHFIELD, D. W. C. (1957) *Brain*, **80**, 293.
SVOLOS, D. G. (1969) *Acta chir. scand.*, Suppl. 401, 1 (Findings in 108 cases).

Plate 38. PITUITARY ADENOMA

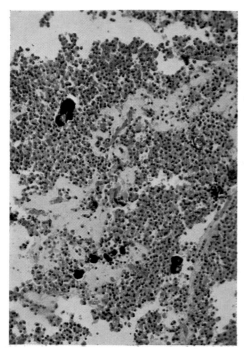

Fig. 1. Calcification of typical chromophobe adenoma. (H & E   × 130)

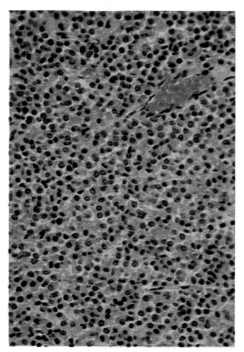

Fig. 2. Chromophobe adenoma composed of solid masses of small regular cells with round nuclei and small amounts of eosinophil cytoplasm. (H & E × 265)

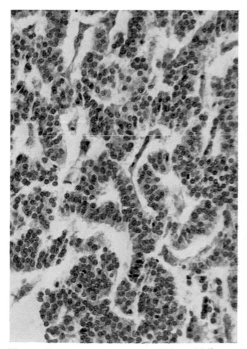

Fig. 3. Chromophobe adenoma of 'sinusoidal' type. (H & E   × 175)

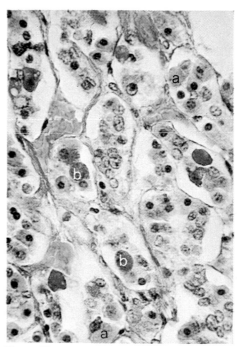

Fig. 4. Normal pituitary cells: acidophils (a) have yellow granules, basophils (b) purple. Chromophobes are agranular. (PAS–Orange G   × 400)

PITUITARY ADENOMA

Case 31. Woman aged 63

History. Six years previously, while in hospital for myocardial infarction, found to have a visual field defect and electrolyte imbalance. Further investigations revealed panhypopituitarism. A non-functioning adenoma was diagnosed. Treatment was effected with yttrium implantation and hormonal replacement. One year progressive deterioration of vision, episodic sleepiness, and headache especially in the morning.

Examination. Hypothyroid appearance with coarse skin and hoarse voice. Visual acuity reduced in left eye (right N6, left N12). Bitemporal visual field defects.

Investigations. Bilateral carotid angiograms showed a suprasellar mass with lateral extensions into the cavernous sinuses, especially on the right.

Operation. Right frontal craniotomy. Tumour had spread up in front of the chiasm from the sella through an opening in the diaphragma 8 mm behind the jugum. There was a large extension of tumour constricted by the two optic nerves lying above the chiasm. A full intracapsular removal of soft, almost diffluent yellowish grey neoplasm was obtained and the tumour capsule disengaged from the thinned chiasm and removed.

Follow-up. Three weeks after operation visual acuity normal (N5) in both eyes. Right visual field full; left superior temporal quadrantic defect persisted.

Microscopical appearances

The tumour is formed of a solid mass of small polyhedral cells with small, regular oval nuclei and sparse, agranular cytoplasm. Mitotic figures are not found. Here and there are cells with clear, unstained cytoplasm. In one or two places there is a sinusoidal pattern of growth where the tumour cells are orientated towards the numerous fine blood-channels.

Diagnosis. Chromophobe adenoma of pituitary.

Summary

Of the adenomas of the anterior pituitary, the chromophobe is the one most often responsible for visual symptoms. In this case the combination of the history, the bitemporal field defects and evidence of hypopituitarism was diagnostic. Following operation, vision was excellent.

The chromophobe adenomas usually present a regular pattern of small, almost uniform, cells in groups intersected by fine blood vessels. Sometimes these appearances can be confused with those of oligodendroglioma or ependymoma: knowledge of the presenting symptoms and the situation of the growth may then be essential for correct interpretation.

Plate 39. PITUITARY ADENOMA

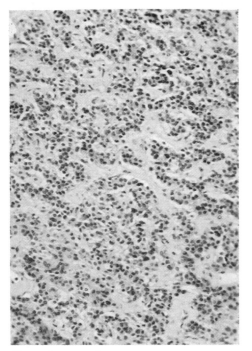

Fig. 1 (Case 31). Chromophobe adenoma. (H & E × 105)

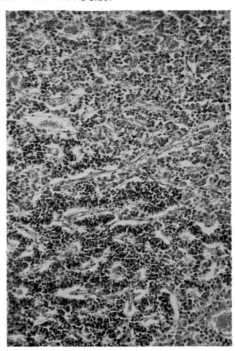

Fig. 2. A minute chromophobe adenoma (sinusoidal type)—a chance finding in a 'normal' pituitary. (H & E × 105)

PITUITARY ADENOMA

Case 32. Woman aged 37

History. Three years previously investigated for amenorrhoea and coarsening of the features with large hands and feet. Left visual field defect covering entire temporal field and lateral third of nasal field. Active acromegaly diagnosed on basis of elevated growth hormone levels. Diabetes mellitus discovered. Air encephalogram (done elsewhere) showed enlargement of the pituitary fossa by a mass with suprasellar extension. Treatment: transnasal yttrium implant. Two months attacks of frontal headache, each lasting about fifteen minutes once a day. Pain was centred on the left side. Diabetes difficult to control.

Examination. Acromegalic. Left eye, proptosis; acuity 6/36; severe field loss in all but the upper nasal quadrant. Right eye normal.

Investigations. Air encephalogram showed the front of the third ventricle to be displaced posteriorly and the tumour to extend above the sella more to the right than the left of the midline. The frontal horns were indented. Carotid angiograms showed an aneurysm of the intracavernous part of the left internal carotid artery, in the vicinity of one of the yttrium rods.

Operation. Right frontal craniotomy. Purple, stringy, vascular tumour within a blue capsule extended from the sella in four directions: along the lesser sphenoid wing on both sides of the sella; forward into the frontal lobe, and upwards through a constriction formed by the anterior cerebral arteries to indent the lamina terminalis and medial aspects of the bodies of the ventricles. A portion of the capsule, adherent to the optic chiasm, had to be left. The left optic nerve was also fused with the growth and its edges could not be defined. In all, about nine-tenths of the mass were removed including the intrasellar portion.

Follow-up. Growth hormone secretion dropped to low level. Diabetes easily controlled.

Microscopical appearances

The tumour is composed of cells that are slightly larger than the typical chromophobe cell, each with a round nucleus containing a prominent nucleolus and a small mass of eosinophil cytoplasm enclosed in a distinct cell membrane. With special staining methods eosinophil cytoplasmic granules can be recognized in many of the cells.

The pattern of growth of the tumour is in solid cellular masses, sometimes intersected by fine capillary blood vessels. There are no malignant features.

Diagnosis. Eosinophil adenoma.

Summary

This patient, a known acromegalic, developed signs indicating extension of a pituitary tumour beyond the sella. As much as possible of the neoplasm was removed, but it could not be separated from the left optic nerve. Microscopically, the tumour was of eosinophil type.

Plate 40. PITUITARY ADENOMA

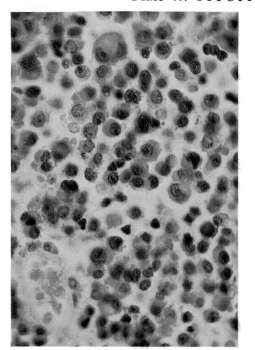

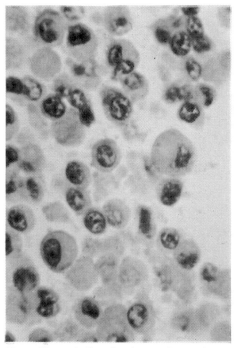

Fig. 1 (Case 32). Eosinophil adenoma. (H & E × 530)

Fig. 2 (Case 32). Cytoplasmic granules are demonstrated by Orange-G. The cells are larger and more globular than chromophobes. (Orange G × 1025)

PITUITARY ADENOMA
Case 33. Woman aged 52

History. Four months' deterioration of vision, particularly in the left eye, pain over left forehead and cheek. Increasing weight and lethargy. Diagnosis of Cushing's syndrome made elsewhere. Given a course of radiotherapy to pituitary fossa.

Examination. Alert and intelligent. Moon-faced. Abdominal striae. 'Buffalo hump'. Blood pressure 180/105. Both optic discs pale. Visual fields: left paracentral scotoma, right normal. No other signs.

Investigations. Endocrine: Plasma 11-hydroxycorticosteroids (average) 60 mg/100 ml; 17-oxogenic 31 mg/24 hours; 17-oxosteroids 9 mg/24 hours. Skull radiograph showed expansion of the sella with destruction of its walls and thinning of the lesser wing of the sphenoid and elevation of the right anterior clinoid indicating lateral displacement of cavernous sinus by tumour. Ventriculogram revealed indentation of the floor of the third ventricle with lateral displacement and elevation of the left temporal horns.

Operation. Right frontal craniotomy. A bluish-red tumour occupied the sella and extended upward, displacing the right optic nerve forwards and also laterally into the right cavernous sinus. The consistency of the growth was tough and fibrous and it was removed piecemeal from the sella and the optic nerve was decompressed. The left optic nerve was not disturbed and the left cavernous sinus not explored.

Follow-up. Postoperatively she was given radiotherapy but the Cushing's syndrome did not improve and two months later a total bilateral adrenalectomy was performed. Two years later her condition was satisfactory and the visual acuity was 6/5 in each eye.

Microscopical appearances
The tumour is composed for the most part of small polyhedral cells with oval nuclei arranged in small acini and sometimes in tubules. Mitotic figures are rare. The majority of the cells contain little stainable cytoplasm. However, there are compact groups of larger cells that contain tiny granules which stain brightly with PAS (basophils).

Diagnosis. Mixed adenoma (chromophobe and basophil).

Summary
A pituitary adenoma with active ACTH secretion was strongly suggested by the clinical history and investigations. At operation the tumour was found extending upward to involve the right optic nerve. Microscopically there were cells of both chromophobe and basophil type.

Plate 41. PITUITARY ADENOMA

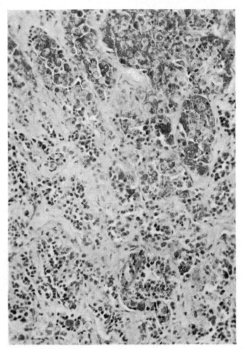

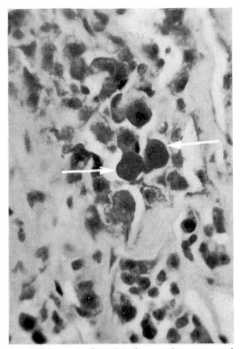

Fig. 1 (Case 33). A mixed population. Groups of large Schiff-positive basophils alternate with chromophobes. (PAS × 105)

Fig. 2 (Case 33). Cytoplasmic granules are strongly Schiff-positive (arrows). (PAS × 630)

CRANIOPHARYNGIOMA
Case 34. Man aged 50

History. Five months' generalized throbbing headache with additional dull, aching right-sided pain. Three months' loss of libido and shaving required less frequently. Four weeks' excessive thirst and polyuria. Three weeks' inability to see to the left with the left eye. He bumped into objects, or people, on the left side.

Examination. Lethargic and obese. Pallor of left optic disc. Visual fields, left homonymous hemianopia (much improved after trial period of steroid therapy). No other abnormality.

Investigations. Endocrine function normal apart from reduction of adrenal function shown by low ketogenic steroids. Skull radiograph normal. Air encephalogram showed a suprasellar mass with indentation of the third ventricle.

Operation. Right frontal craniotomy. Prefixed chiasm behind which pink-grey cystic tumour was seen. Aspiration of the contents produced 2 ml of opalescent fluid, and the cyst wall collapsed and dropped back so that no biopsy was obtainable.

Follow-up. He was well for two months after discharge, and then headaches and visual deterioration, particularly in the left eye, returned. A left paracentral scotoma was found; visual acuity was reduced to 6/24 (left) and 6/12 (right).

Second operation. A right lateral subtemporal approach was used to expose the posterior aspect of the tumour in front of brain stem and behind chiasm. Subtotal removal obtained after aspirating a small cyst without disturbing the floor of the third ventricle.

Progress. Two days following operation the patient's blood pressure fell; on the twelfth day abdominal distension developed and he died. At necropsy there was residual tumour involving the third ventricle and hypothalamic infarction and evidence of acute pancreatitis.

Microscopical appearances

The tumour presents a distinctive pattern formed by trabeculae of squamous epithelial cells alternating with islands of vascular connective tissue and semicystic zones resulting from cellular degeneration. Some cells are of cuboidal or columnar shape, with oval, darkly stained nuclei and tend to be flattened close to masses of keratin; others are larger, paler, polyhedral in outline and have bulky cytoplasm enclosed by a well-defined cell membrane.

Diagnosis. Craniopharyngioma.

Summary

Craniopharyngioma may present with symptoms of visual impairment, or pituitary insufficiency, or with blockage of the third ventricle or with a combination of one or more of these groups. The diagnosis in this case was indicated by the symptomatology and air study, and confirmed at surgery. The technical problems involved in operating on these tumours are often formidable: they may be inseparable from the chiasm and often involve the anterior end of the third ventricle and hypothalamus. In the present case the blood supply to the hypothalamus was implicated. The microscopical features of a partly cystic, epithelial tumour with keratinous masses are typical. Malignant changes have never been described.

These midline tumours are of maldevelopmental origin. They are considered here, rather than with the dermoid and epidermoid cysts, to emphasize their anatomical situation and diagnostic importance in relation to the pituitary gland.

Plate 42. CRANIOPHARYNGIOMA

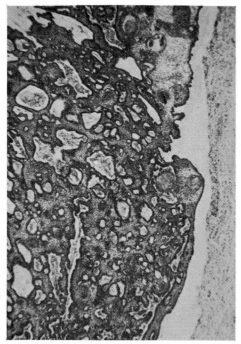

Fig. 1. Craniopharyngioma. An irregular, sieve-like pattern of solid tumour intersected by cysts. (Nissl × 32)

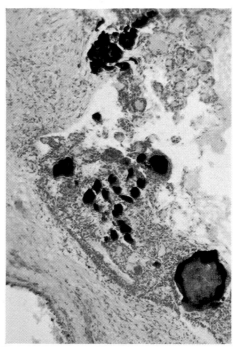

Fig. 2. Calcification of craniopharyngioma. (H & E × 175)

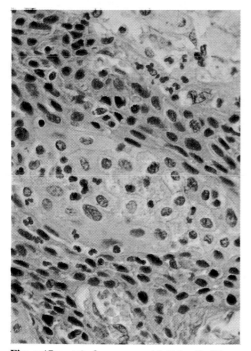

Fig. 3 (Case 34). Squamous epithelial cells (H van Gieson × 420)

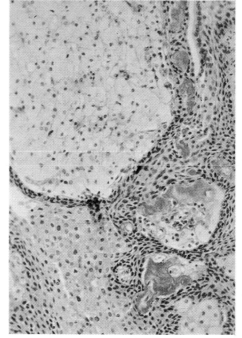

Fig. 4 (Case 34). Cells of immature squamous type forming the lining to a large semicystic pale-staining region. (H van Gieson × 175)

Chordoma

Chordoma is an uncommon tumour, derived from notochordal remnants, which may arise anywhere in the skeleton from the skull to the sacrococcygeal region, with a preference for the midline. Within the cranium the favourite site is the clivus near the spheno-occipital synchondrosis, whence anterior extension of the tumour will involve the pituitary gland and optic chiasm. Pontine compression will result from growth in a posterior direction. Macroscopically the tumour tissue is similar to cartilage—pale blue-grey, semitranslucent and slightly sticky.

Microscopical appearances are of a plentiful mucinous matrix in which lie groups of large polyhedral cells containing multiple vacuoles—the 'physaliphorous' (= 'bubble-bearing') cells,* accompanied by smaller polyhedral cells, signet-ring cells or small spindle cells (Plate 43, Figs. 1, 2).

Chordomas are in essence malignant tumours, frequently recur, and may even produce distant metastases.

Bibliography

CRAWFORD, T. (1958) *J. clin. Path.*, **11,** 110 (Staining reactions).
GESSAGA, E. C., MAIR, W. G. P. and GRANT, D. N. (1973) *Acta neuropath.*, **25,** 27 (Ultrastructure).
STEEGMANN, A. T. (1971) In *Pathology of the Nervous System*, ed. J. Minckler, vol. 2, p. 1917. New York: McGraw-Hill.
STEWART, J. J. and MORRIS, J. E. (1926) *J. Path. Bact.*, **29,** 41.
WILLIS, R. A. (1960) *Pathology of Tumours*, 3rd ed., p. 922. London: Butterworths.

---

* Virchow, who observed small benign gelatinous masses projecting from the clivus and named them ecchondroses' because he believed them to be cartilaginous in origin, used the term 'physaliphora' for the bubbly appearance presented by the cells.

Plate 43. CHORDOMA

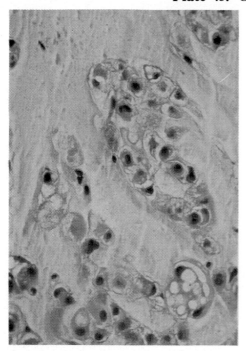

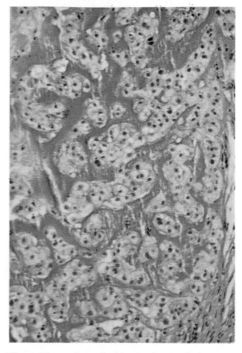

Fig. 1. Clusters of large polyhedral cells, some 'bubble-bearing', in an eosinophil matrix. (H & E × 265)

Fig. 2. Mucopolysaccharides in the matrix between the cords of cells. (Alcian blue × 175)

CHORDOMA
Case 35. Man aged 21

History. Three weeks' only of right-sided headaches. These tended to be episodic, with attacks particularly marked in the morning on waking up, but recurring during the day. Characteristically, a steady ache punctuated with paroxysms of lancinating pain and associated with nausea but not vomiting. The pain had a regular pattern starting in the right orbit, radiating over the forehead down into the subocciput, at times very severe and prostrating.

Examination. No physical signs.

Investigations. Skull radiograph disclosed an erosion of the base of the dorsum sellae but sparing the posterior clinoid and eroding the under-surface of the right anterior clinoidal process. Right carotid arteriogram revealed the pre- and intracavernous portions of the internal carotid artery to be displaced forwards and downwards by an avascular mass. Air encephalogram outlined in an irregular tumour, displacing the lower margin of the third ventricle to the left, projecting into the suprasellar cistern, and laterally displacing the tip of the temporal horn upwards.

Tests of adrenal and thyroid function were normal.

Clinical diagnosis. Probably chordoma, but cholesteatoma and pituitary adenoma were possibilities.

Operation. Right temporal craniotomy with transtemporal approach to the cavernous sinus, the dura of which was bulged laterally. On incision, the very soft, greyish gelatinous contents were intersected by numerous tough septa, typical of a chordoma. The neoplasm extended much further than the radiograph showed, involving the whole of the body of the sphenoid, presumably displacing the third, fourth and sixth nerves upwards, forming irregular pockets in the bone and extending extradurally over the apex of the petrous, down into the posterior fossa. A radical but subtotal removal was obtained, leaving strands infiltrating the bone.

Follow-up. After a course of radiotherapy he was well and free from symptoms and signs apart from fine nystagmus to left and right. Six years later there were no signs of recurrence.

Microscopical appearances

The tumour consists of columns and clumps of large polygonal cells with large vesicular, sometimes vacuolated nuclei. Varying amounts of apparently clear, finely granular or bubbly (physaliphorous) cytoplasm is present. The matrix mucopolysaccharides stain brightly with Alcian blue.

Diagnosis. Chordoma.

Summary

The complete absence of localizing symptoms and signs in this case is notable. It illustrates that there may be very extensive destruction of the base of the skull by tumour without interference with neurological function. The presence of a tumour was only revealed radiologically. Following surgery, progress was excellent, but recurrence must, eventually, be expected. In the majority of these cases repeated recurrences are usual, as it is almost impossible to extirpate these tumours completely.

Plate 44. CHORDOMA

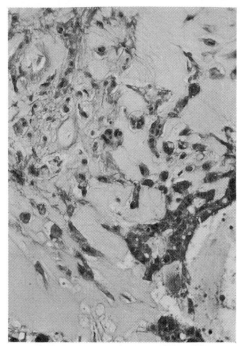

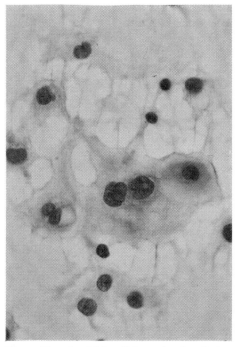

Fig. 1. Columns and small groups of chordoma cells are mostly Schiff-positive; the matrix is faintly stained. (PAS $\times$ 175)

Fig. 2. Vacuolated 'physaliphorous' cells. (H & E $\times$ 530)

Dermoid and epidermoid cysts

Maldevelopmental lesions involving the central nervous system include craniopharyngioma (*see* p. 86), the rare intracranial lipoma, various forms of hamartoma and the more important group of dermoid and epidermoid cysts, which, however, account for only about 2 per cent or less of all intracranial tumours.

Dermoid cysts within the cranial cavity are usually midline, most frequently located in the posterior fossa, and may be connected with the scalp via a sinus, whose discharge may be a useful diagnostic sign. More often these cysts are discovered simply as chronic space-occupying lesions; less commonly meningitis (either bacterial, or chemical from leakage) may be the presenting feature. Spinal dermoids are often lumbosacral in situation and may be associated with syringomyelic cavitation. The lining is of squamous epithelium with some sebaceous glands and hair follicles, and the contents are often dull yellow, thick and cheesy. In the older calcified cysts the lining is frequently defective.

The commoner epidermoid cyst ('cholesteatoma') may be encountered in various intracranial situations: for example the cerebellopontine angle or parapituitary region. These cysts were named '*tumeurs perlées*' by Cruveilhier on account of their pearly opalescent sheen. The lining is a simple flattened layer of squamous epithelium and the contents lamellated keratin (*see* Plate 46, Figs 1, 2). Secondary infection of the contents may lead to the cyst being filled with grumous or frankly purulent material. As with the dermoid cysts, acute or subacute meningitis may be a complication and calcification is well recognized in long-standing cases.

Bibliography

CRITCHLEY, M. and FERGUSON, F. R. (1928) *Brain*, **51**, 334.
LOGUE, V. and TILL, K. (1952) *J. Neurol. Neurosurg. Psychiat.*, **15**, 1.
TAN, T. I. (1972) *Acta neurochir.*, **26**, 13 (Nine cases of epidermoid and three dermoids presented).
TYTUS, J. S. and PENNYBACKER, J. (1956). *J. Neurol Neurosurg. Psychiat.*, **19**, 241.
ULRICH, J. (1964) *J. Neurosurg.*, **21**, 1051 (Seven cases of epidermoid cyst described).

Plate 45. DERMOID AND EPIDERMOID CYSTS

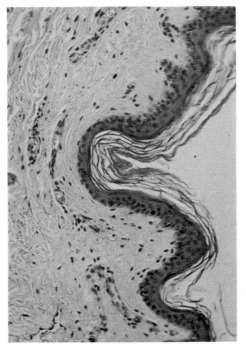

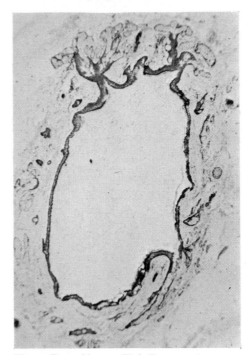

Fig. 1. Normal skin. The squamous epithelium is keratinized. (H & E   × 105)

Fig. 2. Dermoid cyst. (H & E   × 26)

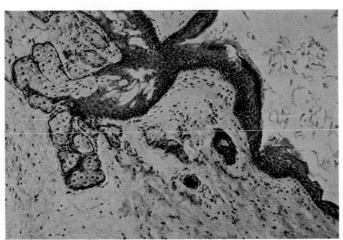

Fig. 3. The lining of the dermoid cyst includes sebaceous glands. (H & E × 105)

EPIDERMOID CYST
Case 36. Woman aged 61

History. Loss of vision in left eye for many years. Two attacks of transient visual disturbance in the right eye, each lasting about thirty minutes, eight years previously. Progressive loss of vision in right eye for one year.

Examination. Left eye, cataract. Acuity, counting fingers at 1 m. Right eye, visual acuity 6/24. Bitemporal visual field defect with main emphasis in upper quadrants. Pallor of right optic disc.

Investigations. Carotid angiograms showed a small aneurysm of the anterior communicating artery. Right vertebral angiogram normal. Air encephalogram revealed elevation of the anterior end of the third ventricle and posterior displacement of the aqueduct and fourth ventricle. A mass was outlined above the posterior half of the sella.

Operation. Right frontal craniotomy. The right side of the chiasm was adherent to the capsule of a mass of glistening white cholesteatoma with a large subfrontal extension. A solid nubbin lay to the right side of the jugum, on top of the right optic nerve and running behind and beneath it. The chiasm was displaced downwards and backwards. The bulk of the tumour, with its capsule, was removed from round the chiasm and optic nerves but dense adhesions between the right optic nerve and the capsule prevented total removal. The right optic nerve appeared attenuated; the left healthy.

Follow-up. Post operative visual acuity in the right eye was reduced to recognizing hand movements. After operation for cataract vision in the left eye improved to 6/9. Three years later there was no sign of recurrent tumour and vision was unchanged.

Microscopical appearances

The cyst membrane is tortuous and is composed of simple squamous epithelium resting on collagenous tissue. Abundant lamellated keratin is found within the cyst.

Diagnosis. Epidermoid cyst (cholesteatoma).

Summary

This patient presented with slowly progressive visual loss in one eye, with a suprasellar mass revealed on air study. Diagnostic possibilities were meningioma, pituitary adenoma or developmental cyst: at operation the nature of the mass was revealed.

Epidermoids are typically encapsulated, glistening cystic tumours which may be found in a variety of intracranial situations. Their contents are extremely irritant, and may cause chemical meningitis if disseminated by spontaneous, or operative, rupture.

Plate 46. EPIDERMOID CYST

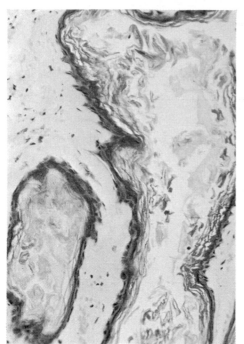

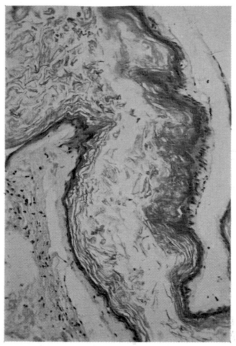

Fig. 1 (Case 36). Lamellated keratin is present within the cyst. The lining is a simple layer of epithelium with no appendages. (H & E × 130)

Fig. 2. The epithelial layer is incomplete in some places. (H & E × 130)

x

Tumours of meninges

MENINGIOMA

The great majority of meningiomas are benign tumours. Their mode of growth is expansive; they compress but do not infiltrate the brain or cord. Their microscopical appearances are seldom atypical. Intracranial meningiomas are much commoner than intraspinal; in Cushing's series the proportion was sixteen to one. Within the skull these tumours are usually found attached to the dura mater in relation to the venous sinuses and the commonest situations are parasagittal, sphenoidal ridge, olfactory groove, parasellar and petrous temporal. The intraventricular choroid plexus meningioma, and the diffuse thickening without a large mass 'meningioma *en plaque*' are less common. A small proportion of meningiomas are associated with hyperostosis cranii (4·5 per cent of Cushing and Eisenhardt's cases).

The naked-eye appearances of these tumours is characteristic; they are frequently purple-grey in colour, firm and gritty in texture, less commonly pale grey and relatively avascular, or soft and yellow from fat storage.

Their microscopical appearances have been classified in various ways (Cushing and Eisenhardt 1938; Russell and Rubinstein 1971) but, in general, these histological subdivisions have no prognostic significance and in many examples the appearances vary considerably in different areas. But, as a practical matter of recognition certain distinct types can be recognized. The tumours often possess oval, vesicular, sometimes vacuolated nuclei disposed in a regular manner in a simple matrix. This is the basis of the 'syncytial' or 'endotheliomatous' or 'meningotheliomatous' type of growth. There is no sharp demarcation between this pattern and the tumours in which whorl-formation is prominent. Here the cells tend to be wrapped round each other often with a small vessel at the centre of the 'whorl' (*see* Plate 48, Figs 1, 2). When calcium salts are laid down in the whorl 'psammoma bodies' are formed. The terms 'psammomatous' or 'whorling' meningioma are sometimes employed. More convenient perhaps is the term 'transitional' meningioma when used for meningiomas with conspicuous whorl formation that are regarded as 'transitional' between the syncytial and the fibroblastic type.

In the 'fibroblastic' type the cells are elongated and spindle-shaped, running in thick bundles, sometimes with associated whorl-formations. Fine connective tissue fibres are often plentiful (*see* Plate 50, Figs 1, 2).

The rare angioblastic type of meningioma includes two distinct patterns of growth (Pitkethly et al. 1973). In the first, the appearances are similar to those of the haemangioblastoma of the cerebellum. The second is the haemangiopericytic type, similar to the haemangiopericytoma occurring elsewhere in the body, and characterized by closely packed cells with curved or oval nuclei and sparse cytoplasm which abut on capillary blood spaces, which may be dilated, or compressed and consequently inconspicuous (*see* Plate 47, Fig. 1). A reticulin impregnation may be helpful in outlining these channels. The incidence of mitotic division is often higher than in the commoner types of meningioma and a rapid tempo of growth is indicated by frequent recurrences. A careful distinction

Plate 47. MENINGIOMA

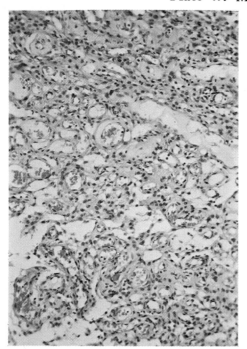

Fig. 1. Syncytial meningioma containing numerous dilated blood vessels. This angiomatoid appearance is often interpreted as 'angioblastic'. (H & E × 105)

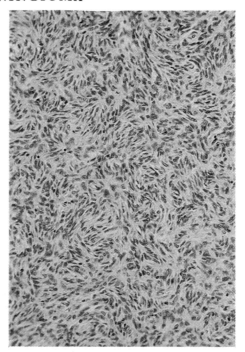

Fig. 2. Angioblastic meningioma of the type resembling haemangiopericytoma. Cells with elongated or oval nuclei are disposed in close relation to capillary blood vessels, many of which are compressed and inconspicuous. (H & E × 175)

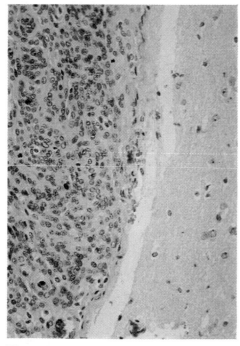

Fig. 3. Edge of a 'typical' meningioma. (H & E × 210)

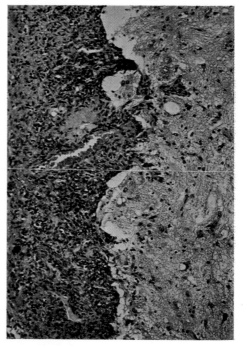

Fig. 4. Malignant meningioma. There is no capsule. Short tongues of tumour penetrate gliotic brain tissue. (H & E × 105)

must be made between the true angioblastic meningiomas and the much commoner situation of a syncytial meningioma containing very numerous blood vessels with a resulting 'angiomatoid' appearance.

Foamy cells laden with fat may be a feature of meningiomas ('xanthomatous' type). Bone may be present, particularly in the spinal meningiomas (*see* Plate 51, Fig. 2) and, much more rarely, cartilage.

Malignant changes

The typical microscopical appearance of a meningioma is not always a reliable sign of a good prognosis. The problem of recurrence along the dura into the sinuses is a common and important one in neurosurgical practice, but often arises with entirely 'typical' tumours. Conversely, such apparently sinister features as giant cells (*see* Plate 49, Fig. 3) mitotic figures and necrotic foci, usually associated with rapidity of growth and infiltrative capacity, may be found in meningiomas whose behaviour exemplifies 'benignity'. In all cases examination of the edges of the growth should be carefully carried out whenever possible, for the presence of finger-like projections of tumour into gliotic brain substance is an important sign of enhanced malignancy and extensive involvement of the outlying dura points to the probability of recurrence.

The angioblastic meningioma has been cited as the histological variety most commonly associated with malignancy (*see* Plate 47, Fig. 4).

Extracranial metastases of meningioma are very rare and may be slow-growing. In some recorded cases a papillary architecture developed in the secondary tumour (Cushing and Eisenhardt 1938).

SARCOMA

Involvement of the nervous system and its coverings by sarcoma is rare. When the malignant meningiomas, the lymphoreticular group of tumours, and the medulloblastomas extending into the leptomeninges ('arachnoidal sarcoma', *see* p. 60), are put on one side a small group of neoplasms arising from connective tissue elements remains. Polymorphic sarcoma in the brain is a well recognized, if rare, tumour of infancy. Meningeal fibrosarcomas arising from the dura or from the leptomeninges may be found in adults and their microscopical appearances are usually similar to those of sarcomas elsewhere in the body (*see* Plate 53, Fig. 1). Kernohan and Uihlein (1962) point out that the prognosis in these neoplasms is very variable: some fibrosarcomas are relatively slow-growing. Myxosarcoma and chondrosarcoma of the meninges have been described, but are rare.

MELANOMA

Primary melanoma of the meninges may take the form of a localized tumour or a diffuse widespread infiltration. The growth is believed to originate from pigmented cells normally present in the pia. Behaviour is usually that of a highly malignant tumour. The diagnosis can only be made with certainty after a careful post-mortem examination in which all possible primary sites of melanoma—eyes, skin, viscera, nail-beds—are excluded. A pigmented meningioma or Schwannoma may sometimes be mistaken for a melanoma but usually the characteristic appearances of these tumours enable them to be identified correctly.

Bibliography

Meningioma

BAKAY, L. and CARES, H. L. (1972) *Acta neurochir.*, **26,** 1 (Twenty-five cases of olfactory groove meningioma).

CERVOS-NAVARRO, J. and VAZQUEZ, J. J. (1969) *Acta neuropath.*, **13,** 301 (Ultrastructure).

CUSHING, H. and EISENHARDT, LOUISE (1938) *Meningiomas*. Springfield, Ill.: Charles C Thomas (Contains a wealth of information and illustration).

EARLE, K. M. and RICHANY, S. F. (1969) *Med. Ann. D.C.*, **38,** 353.

EL-BANHAWY, A., SHELDON, P. W. E. and PENNYBACKER, J. (1963) *J. Neurol. Neurosurg. Psychiat.*, **26,** 462 ('On missing meningiomas').

KEPES, J. (1961) *Am. J. Path.*, **39,** 499 (Ultrastructure).

PITKETHLY, D. T., HARDMAN, J. M., KEMPE, L. C. and EARLE, K. M. (1970) *J. Neurosurg.*, **32,** 539 (A study of eighty-one angioblastic meningiomas).

RUSSELL, DOROTHY S. and RUBINSTEIN, L. J. (1971). See p. x.

TYTUS, J. S., LASERSOHN, J. T. and REIFEL, E. (1967) *J. Neurosurg.*, **27,** 551 (Discussion of malignancy).

Sarcoma

KERNOHAN, J. W. and UIHLEIN, A. (1962) *Sarcomas of the Brain*. Springfield, Ill.: Charles C Thomas.

RUBINSTEIN, L. J. (1971) In *Pathology of the Nervous System*, ed. J. Minckler, vol. 2, p. 2144. New York: McGraw-Hill.

Melanoma

GIBSON, J. B., BURROWS, D. and WEIR, W. P. (1957) *J. Path. Bact.*, **74,** 419.

MENINGIOMA
Case 37. Woman aged 62

History. Seven years' gradual loss of vision in right eye. Seven months' progressive loss of vision in left eye. At first she noticed that she was not seeing so well on the left side, then her sight deteriorated to the point at which she could only read the newspaper headlines. Six months before admission developed hyperthyroidism. Weight reduced by 20 kg (40 lb). Treated medically. Weight regained.

Examination. Mental functions all normal. Ocular fundi: bilateral atrophy. Right eye totally blind. Left eye, visual acuity 6/60. Left temporal field defect; nasal field full. No pyramidal deficit. Skin pale, pubic and axillary hair sparse.

Investigations. Skull radiograph revealed that the pituitary fossa was not enlarged. There was dense opacity involving the bone of the jugum sphenoidale and root of the lesser wing of the right sphenoid and anterior border of the sella turcica. Scintiscan showed doubtful increased uptake above and to the right of the pituitary fossa. Carotid angiograms showed the mass to be centred on the tuberculum sellae extending to the right of the midline. It was supplied by meningeal branches derived from the ophthalmic arteries.

Clinical diagnosis. Meningioma likely.

Operation. Right frontal craniotomy. A pinkish grey tumour was attached to the dura mater over the jugum sphenoidale extending forwards for about 2 cm to reach to within 1 cm of the posterior margin of the crista galli. The right optic nerve could not be identified and clearly was incorporated in the mass. As much as possible was removed but some tumour tissue adherent to the left optic nerve had to be left.

Follow-up. Following the operation a small amount of vision returned to the temporal field of the right eye and acuity in the left eye improved to N24. Three years later she felt well and had no fresh neurological symptoms.

Microscopical appearances

The tumour cells are of regular size with oval, often vacuolated nuclei. They lie in a syncytial mass in which cell outlines are indistinct. In some places whorl-formation is present: in these structures the cells are wrapped one around the next to form a rounded mass that is sometimes calcified. Blood vessels are sparse. Mitotic figures are not found.

Diagnosis. Meningioma of syncytial type.

Summary

The history of gradual visual deterioration affecting first one eye, then the other, with evidence of a mass at the jugum with bony involvement, strongly suggested meningioma. Despite the incomplete removal useful vision was obtained and the growth has not recurred.

Microscopically this is a typical example of the commonest type of meningioma: syncytial masses of cells with whorl formation ('syncytial' or 'transitional' type).

Plate 48. MENINGIOMA

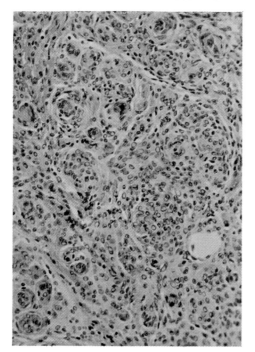

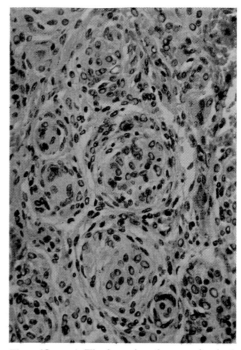

Fig. 1 (Case 37). The tumour is composed of cells with oval, often vacuolated, nuclei of regular shape and size. (H & E × 175)

Fig. 2 (Case 37). The formation of concentric whorls is frequent. (H & E × 265)

MENINGIOMA
Case 38. Man aged 50

History. Eight weeks' attacks of transient weakness of the right leg and inability to move the right foot associated with dizziness, each lasting one to two minutes. Seven days' mild headaches once or twice a day each lasting five to ten minutes, no vomiting.

Examination. Facial asymmetry due to right upper motor neuron facial paresis; no other signs.

Investigations. Skull radiograph showed enlargement of the left foramen spinosum. Electro-encephalograph appearances suggested a left frontal structural lesion. Left carotid angiogram revealed a left frontal expanding lesion with no pathological circulation. Ventriculograms confirmed a large left frontal mass with backward displacement and indentation of the frontal horn and body of the ventricle. The appearances suggested an infiltrative glioma.

Operation. Left frontal craniotomy. Soft purple tumour tissue extruded through the dura from an attachment about 5 cm across over the posterior aspect of the left frontal sinus. It had indented the frontal lobe. After evacuation of the central part of the tumour the capsule was dissected completely from the brain leaving a cavity 6 cm in diameter.

Follow-up. During the first seven days following operation there were signs of right hemi-paresis and expressive dysphasia which cleared completely. He made a full recovery and resumed a distinguished academic career. Fifteen years later he was in excellent health.

Microscopical appearances

The cells of the tumour are arranged in sheets and loose whorls. The cytoplasm is uniformly clear and pale-staining throughout the tumour. The individual cells are polygonal and vary markedly in size. Some nuclei are small and elliptical, others very large and oval; many contain vacuoles. Collagen is sparse. Some small portions of tumour are necrotic. Mitoses are not seen.

Diagnosis. Syncytial meningioma, but of unusual cellular pleomorphism.

Summary

The short history of symptoms in this case, coupled with the ventriculographic appearances, favoured a glioma. However, at operation the growth was firmly attached to the dura and could be dissected cleanly from the brain. The postoperative course was (and is) highly satisfactory.

At the time of the initial pathological examination the presence of giant cells and necrotic foci was viewed with some disquiet, though the tumour was, of course, considered generally benign. In a minority of meningiomas, cellular polymorphism of this degree must be accepted as within the normal range of appearances.

Plate 49. MENINGIOMA

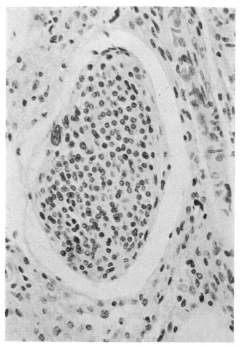

Fig. 1 (Case 38). A group of cells of regular appearance. (H & E × 265)

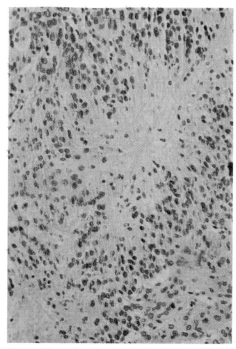

Fig. 2 (Case 38). Necrosis in the tumour. (H & E × 175)

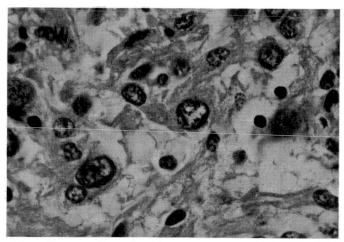

Fig. 3 (Case 38). Giant cells with abundant nuclear chromatin. (H & E × 660)

MENINGIOMA
Case 39. Woman aged 46

History. Fourteen weeks' episodic bouts of headache, becoming more frequent and persistent, some associated with vomiting. Four weeks' blurring of vision and periods of double vision on looking straight ahead; unsteady gait observed by friends.

Examination. Drowsy, but mental functions normal. Marked bilateral papilloedema. Visual acuity reduced, 6/12 right and left, blind spots enlarged. Nystagmus on looking to the right. Ataxia of left hand and slight ataxia of gait. Limb reflexes sluggish but symmetrical.

Investigations. Left carotid angiogram normal. Scintiscan showed increased uptake in the posterior fossa on the left side. Ventriculograms revealed dilatation of the lateral and third ventricles and displacement of the fourth ventricle to the right by a left-sided mass.

Operation. Left suboccipital craniotomy. The dura mater was discoloured and abnormally vascular and a firm lump felt at a depth of 4 cm by needling. Opening the dura a large reddish-grey encapsulated tumour occupying almost the whole of the lateral half of the left cerebellar hemisphere was displayed. It was attached to the dura mater posterosuperiorly, adjacent to the lateral sinus. It was completely excised.

Follow-up. Excellent recovery; reported very well six years later.

Microscopical appearances

The tumour is a dense growth of thin spindle-shaped cells arranged in large interlacing bundles. The nuclei are ovoid, vesicular and tend to be uniform. Reticulin impregnations demonstrate fine connective tissue fibrils between the cells.

Diagnosis. Meningioma of fibroblastic type.

Summary

The symptoms and signs, together with results of special investigations, pointed to a posterior fossa tumour. An encapsulated meningioma was found and removed with excellent results. It presented the appearances of bundles of spindle cells, with numerous intercellular connective tissue fibrils. This fibroblastic type of meningioma is well-recognized in many situations: it is said that the majority of intraventricular meningiomas are fibroblastic.

Plate 50. MENINGIOMA

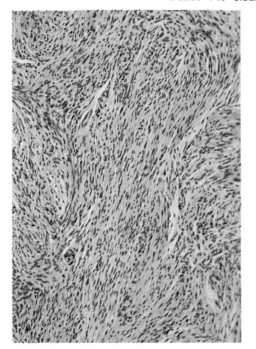

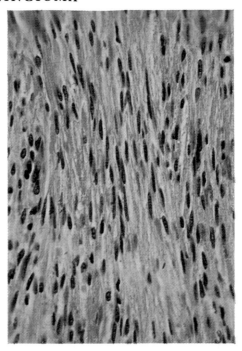

Fig. 1 (Case 39). Closely packed bundles of thin spindle cells with oval nuclei. (H & E   × 105)

Fig. 2 (Case 39). Elongated cells of fibroblastic type. (H & E   × 420)

MENINGIOMA
Case 40. Woman aged 77

History. Two years previously, B12-deficiency anaemia diagnosed and treated; no neurological signs at that time. Nine months' progressive paraesthesiae and weakness of both legs; both feet completely numb. Two months' unable to walk at all; sensory loss affecting both legs, two burns of left leg.

Examination. Mentally normal. Loss of sensation to all modalities below L1. Spastic paraparesis affecting right leg more than left. Bladder function normal.

Investigations. Lumbar puncture revealed a partial manometric block. Lumbar myelogram showed a block at D12 and cisternal myelogram disclosed the upper level of the block 2 cm higher.

Operation. Thoracic laminectomy D10, 11, 12. A firm rounded tumour 2 cm in diameter and 1·5 cm thick was seen on opening the dura, lying on the right lateral and posterior aspect of the cord, involving the root exits of the sensory and motor branches of D11 on the right, which were cut. The tumour, with its capsule intact, was removed with attached dura.

Follow-up. Two weeks after operation there was a steady return of power to both legs and sensation to pin-prick had returned. Six years later (aged 83) she was able to get about, walking normally, and had no complaints.

Microscopical appearances

The tumour is highly cellular, formed of cells with oval or spindle-shaped vesicular nuclei that sometimes are vacuolated. There are no clear cell margins. The arrangement is in wide bundles, solid syncytial masses or whorls and there are numerous lamellated psammoma bodies in which calcium salts are deposited. In one region there is conspicuous formation of mature bone.

Diagnosis. Psammomatous meningioma with bone formation.

Summary

In this elderly woman the history of B12-deficiency raised the possibility of subacute combined degeneration of the spinal cord. However, it was soon evident that this was a case of cord compression due to tumour. Removal of the meningioma produced a satisfactory result.

Bone formation in meningiomas was noted by Cushing and Eisenhardt (1938). They used the term 'osteoblastic meningioma' for such tumours and regarded them as rare (of the order of 1 per cent).

Plate 51. MENINGIOMA

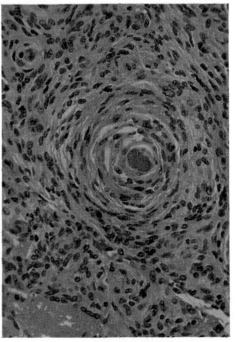

Fig. 1 (Case 40). Meningioma with calcified psammoma body. Many nuclei are vacuolated. (H & E
× 210)

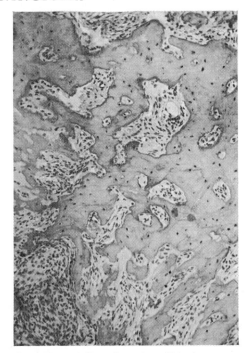

Fig. 2 (Case 40). Bone formation within the tumour.
(H & E   × 105)

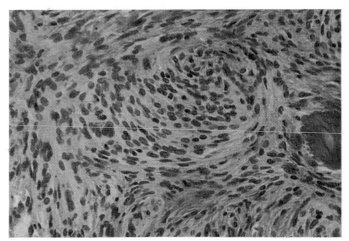

Fig. 3 (Case 40). Cells with oval nuclei arranged in whorl formation.
(H & E   × 210)

MENINGIOMA
Case 41. Woman aged 51

History. Several weeks' mental deterioration. For some years she had been 'a bit strange'; now she had quietly become confused and vacant, and developed urinary incontinence. Four days' severe left-sided headaches with nausea and vomiting; one episode of loss of consciousness for a few minutes, but no frank convulsion.

Examination. Disorientated in time and space; uncommunicative and unable to give a history. Apathetic and inert. Bilateral papilloedema. Limb reflexes brisk but symmetrical. Left plantar response extensor.

Investigations. Skull radiographs showed decalcification of the posterior clinoid processes. Carotid angiograms revealed the presence of a large tumour in the left frontal region with fine pathological vessels indicative of a meningioma supplied from the external carotid meningeal branches.

Operation. Bilateral frontal craniotomy. A large bilateral frontal parasagittal meningioma was found, with a left frontal exostosis. It was attached to the falx over about 9 cm and extended from just above the crista galli to the level of the coronal suture. The main mass was on the left but a large nubbin extended laterally under the right frontal cortex. It was almost completely excised, with the falx and the obstructed sagittal sinus, but the left prerolandic cortical veins ran through the posterior margin of the mass, and here some growth had to be left.

Follow-up. Immediate recovery excellent. Six months later readmitted with large bilateral recurrence, mainly on the right side. The tumour was again removed and she was given a course of radiotherapy. Six months later again she returned with a large left frontal recurrence, with infiltration of the cranium and two subcutaneous extensions from the bone, and died.

Necropsy. Soft tumour occupied much of the left frontal lobe. It replaced the falx and fungated through the craniotomy site to infiltrate the scalp. No extracranial organs were involved.

Microscopical appearances

First operation. The overall appearance is typical meningioma (Plate 52, Fig. 1). The tumour cells are of fairly uniform size with oval nuclei and indistinct outlines tending to be arranged in compact bundles and whorls, with a few psammoma bodies. Rarely, groups of larger cells with bulky eosinophil cytoplasm are found.

Recurrence and post-mortem. There is considerable change in the appearance of the tumour (Plate 52, Fig. 2). Cellular pleomorphism is striking, with a high proportion of giant cells with multiple nuclei or very large single nuclei with coarse nuclear chromatin, and substantial eosinophil cytoplasm. Mitotic figures are present. Whorl formation is not evident. In many places the tumour is necrotic and infiltrated with lymphocytes. There is an extensive fibrovascular network.

Diagnosis. Meningioma (malignant).

Summary
The progressively malignant course of this tumour, shown both clinically and pathologically, is fortunately rare.

Plate 52. MENINGIOMA

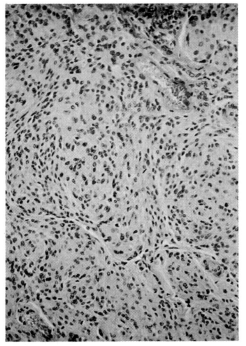

Fig. 1 (Case 41). First biopsy. Typical meningioma.
(H & E   × 175)

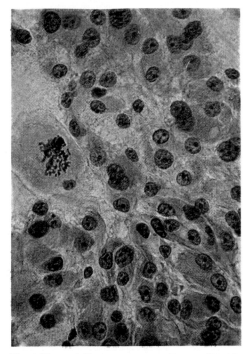

Fig. 2 (Case 41). Recurrent tumour. Large cells with
bulky eosinophil cytoplasm and prominent nucleoli.
One cell in mitosis. (H & E   × 420)

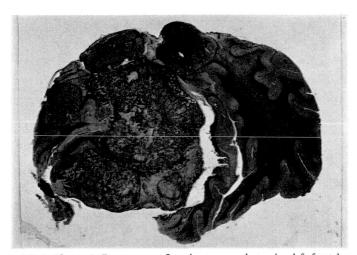

Fig. 3 (Case 41). Post-mortem. Invasive tumour destroying left frontal
lobe. PTAH   × 0.37)

MENINGEAL SARCOMA
Case 42. Woman aged 55

History. Six months previously, one attack of momentary loss of consciousness followed by progressive change in personality. She became slow, forgetful, apathetic and inactive. Three weeks' difficulty with words, 'cannot express herself' and noted to be using wrong names. Difficulty in dressing herself. Ten days' staggering from side to side and tending to fall down. Several episodes of headache but no spontaneous complaint. Incontinent.

Examination. Drowsy, disorientated and unsteady. Understood simple commands but marked expressive and receptive dysphasia. Bilateral papilloedema. Right lower motor neuron facial weakness. Knee and ankle jerks exaggerated on both sides. Bilateral extensor plantar responses.

Investigations. Electroencephalograph abnormalities suggested a deep left frontal tumour. Left carotid angiogram showed a characteristic shift of the anterior cerebral artery 1 cm to the right indicative of a frontal tumour.

Operation. Rock-hard, avascular tumour was attached to the parasagittal dura and to the falx extending to both left and right sides. The centre of the growth was removed and the capsule stripped from the dura with little bleeding.

Follow-up. Rapid improvement followed a course of radiotherapy. Three months later dysphasia was only very slight and she had returned to her normal activities. Eight months later she deteriorated with dysphasia and hemiparesis but angiograms did not disclose a localized recurrence. She died a year later.

Microscopical appearances

A large portion of the tumour is necrotic. The more cellular viable zones are made up of spindle-shaped cells whose oval nuclei contain clumped nuclear chromatin and prominent eosinophil nucleoli. Fine collagen fibres are abundant, mitotic figures are numerous. Endothelial proliferation of blood vessels is marked, with fibrous vascular occlusion.

Diagnosis. Spindle-cell sarcoma of meninges.

Summary

Primary fibrosarcoma of the meninges resembles fibrosarcoma in other parts of the body and carries a poor prognosis. It is a rare tumour in adults, rather more common in childhood. The microscopical picture is of elongated spindle cells associated with a rich network of connective tissue fibrils; mitotic figures are numerous and the centre of the growth may be necrotic. At the edges tongues of invading tumour penetrate the nervous tissue, often stimulating a very marked reaction on the part of the astrocytes. In some cases, usually those with a long clinical history, the appearances suggest sarcomatous evolution of a meningioma, in others (such as the present one) the neoplasm shows no sign of a pre-existing benign lesion.

Plate 53. MENINGEAL SARCOMA

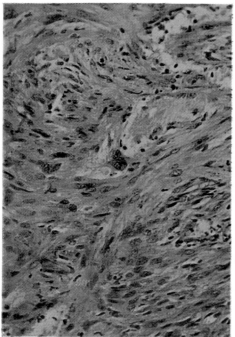

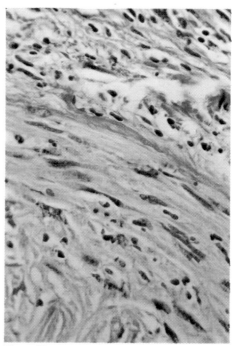

Fig. 1 (Case 42). Bundles of irregular spindle cells with pleomorphic nuclei. (H & E × 265)

Fig. 2 (Case 42). Tumour cells with elongated and triangular nuclei in a bundle with a collagenous matrix. (H van Gieson × 420)

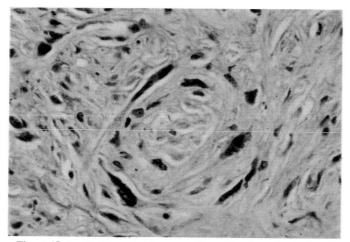

Fig. 3 (Case 42). Elongated tumour cells within the wall of a blood vessel. (H van Gieson × 420)

MENINGEAL MELANOMA

Case 43. Man aged 30

History. Eight months' headache, at first intermittent, then becoming increasingly severe, and for three to four months continuous. It was mainly frontal and bilateral, but sometimes extended to the occipital regions. Two months' vomiting, increasing in frequency from once a week to every day. For two days headache and vomiting much worse.

Examination. Mental functions normal. Severe bilateral papilloedema with haemorrhages and exudates. Left ptosis. Slight right hemiparesis and bilateral extensor plantar responses.

Investigations. Skull radiograph revealed erosion of the sella turcica. Scintiscan showed a dense area of increased uptake in the middle fossa suggesting meningioma. Left carotid angiogram revealed a large middle and anterior temporal mass lying superficially with supply from middle meningeal and superficial temporal arteries with capillary 'blush'.

Operation. Left temporal craniotomy. The dura mater was darkly discoloured and in places black. A large tumour was attached to the dura covering the floor and lateral wall of the temporal fossa in front of the petrous ridge. Anteriorly it was jet-black; posteriorly it was pale grey-brown. It could be dissected from the underlying brain and was removed completely with its capsule. The discoloured dura was partly removed but had to be left in the region of the pterion.

Follow-up. Following the operation he was free of symptoms and the papilloedema subsided. There was no sign of cutaneous or ocular melanoma.

Microscopical appearances

The tumour is composed of solid masses of large polygonal cells with spheroidal nuclei containing conspicuous nucleoli and with clearly defined cytoplasm, sometimes pale, sometimes dark brown. This pigment reacts with the Masson–Fontana method for melanin. Mitotic figures are fairly numerous. In places there is sharp demarcation between pigmented and non-pigmented tumour. There is no demonstrable infiltration of brain. In the dura mater there are small outlying foci of pigmented tumour, and in addition there are small elevated nodules formed of proliferating fibroblasts each with small numbers of pigment-bearing cells at the base of the nodule.

Diagnosis. Melanoma of the dura. The histological appearances, together with the lack of demonstrable cutaneous or visceral lesions, suggest that it is a primary tumour.

Summary

The history and investigations suggested a benign meningioma, but at operation extensive black discoloration of the dura mater and partial black coloration of the tumour substance, were noted. The microscopical appearances are clearly those of melanoma. In this case, as in others, the diagnosis of a 'primary' melanoma must remain presumptive, unless a full *post mortem* study reveals no cutaneous (or visceral) primary.

Plate 54. MENINGEAL MELANOMA

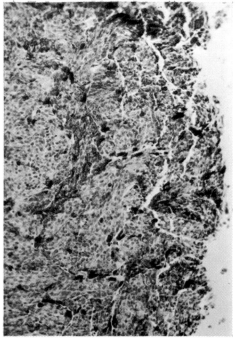

Fig. 1 (Case 43). Brown or black pigmentation of a high proportion of tumour cells. (H & E   × 130)

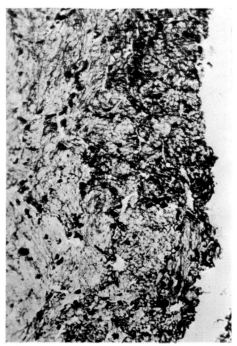

Fig. 2 (Case 43). With Fontana's method the melanin-bearing cells are impregnated black. (Fontana   × 130)

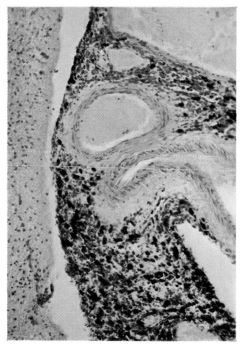

Fig. 3. Pigmented melanoma cells in leptomeninges. (Fontana   × 105)

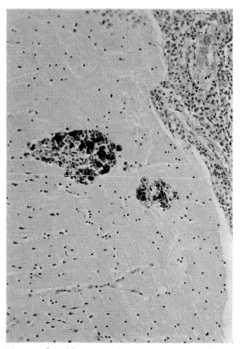

Fig. 4. In this case of primary leptomeningeal melanoma pigmented cells are penetrating the cortex from the distended Virchow–Robin spaces. The meningeal tumour is not pigmented. (H & E × 105)

Tumours of nerve roots: Schwannoma and neurofibroma

The nomenclature for this group of tumours is both varied and confusing. Some authorities do not separate the two types of tumour under discussion.

The term 'Schwannoma' is used for those common neoplasms of cranial and spinal roots sometimes known as neurinomas or neurilemmomas. These tumours are encapsulated and consist of a compact proliferation of bundles of elongated spindle-cells with plump oval nuclei, often ranged in 'palisade' formation, alternating with regions of looser-textured tissue in which the cells are comparatively sparse and which may become cystic (Plate 55, Fig. 1; *see also* Plate 56, Fig. 2). They are rich in reticulin fibres, and usually devoid of axons. In the 'neurofibroma' (Plate 55, Fig. 2), smaller cells with narrow nuclei are sparsely distributed in a collagenous matrix, and the axons belonging to the nerve from which the growth arises can often be found, though probably split and fragmented, within its substance (Plate 55, Fig. 3).

In multiple neurofibromatosis (von Recklinghausen's disease) tumours of both types may be found. In addition there may be gliomas of the optic nerve or brain (often midline, see Case 3), meningiomas, ependymomas, phaeochrome tumours of the adrenal medulla, and, of course, the well-known skin lesions. Malignant change is rare in Schwannoma or neurofibroma, and when it occurs, is usually in cases of von Recklinghausen's disease. This is in contrast with the findings in experimental tumour induction using the N-nitroso compounds: in these circumstances malignant Schwannomas are common.

Bibliography

CRAVIOTO, H. (1969) *Acta neuropath.*, **12**, 116 (Fine structure of acoustic neuroma).

CUSHING, H. (1917) *Tumors of the Nervus Acusticus and the Syndrome of Cerebellopontile Angle.* Philadelphia: Saunders.

EDWARDS, C. H. and PATERSON, J. H. (1951) *Brain*, **74**, 144 (Symptoms and signs analysed in 157 unilateral and seven bilateral acoustic tumours).

GAUTIER-SMITH, P. C. (1967) *Brain*, **90**, 359 (Clinical aspects of spinal neurofibromas).

HARKIN, J. C. and REED, R. J. (1969) *Tumors of the Peripheral Nervous System. Atlas of Tumor Pathology*, Second Series, Fascicle 3. Washington, D.C.: Armed Forces Institute of Pathology.

RUSSELL, DOROTHY S. and RUBINSTEIN, L. J. (1971) See p. x.

SLOOFF, J. L., KERNOHAN, J. W. and MACCARTY, C. S. (1964) See p. x.

Plate 55. SCHWANNOMA AND NEUROFIBROMA

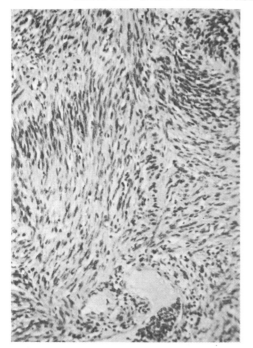

Fig. 1. Schwannoma. Bundles of elongated spindle-cells whose nuclei are aligned in parallel ('palisading'). (H & E   × 105)

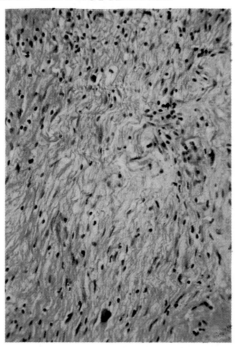

Fig. 2. Neurofibroma. Fibroblasts with elongated oval nuclei, and small cells with rounded nuclei, in a connective tissue matrix. (H van Gieson   × 130)

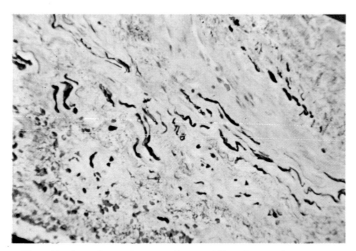

Fig. 3. Portions of axons in a neurofibroma. (Glees-Marsland   × 210)

SCHWANNOMA
Case 44. Woman aged 49

History. Nine months' deafness of right ear, with an abnormal 'rushing noise'. Three months' attacks of headache with nausea and vomiting. Four weeks' unsteady walking, developed aching pain localized to the right ear, aggravated by coughing and sneezing. One week's rapid deterioration in balance, unable to stand without help.

Examination. Mentally dull and very forgetful. Could not attempt serial seven test. Bilateral papilloedema. Right corneal reflex absent. Severe deafness of right ear; left normal, no facial weakness. Slight ataxia of lower limbs in heel to knee to shin test but gait very unsteady and Romberg's sign present.

Investigations. Skull radiographs showed enlargement and erosion of the sella turcica and enlargement of the right internal auditory meatus. Right carotid angiogram revealed symmetrical hydrocephalus. Vertebral angiogram disclosed a right cerebellopontine angle tumour about 3·5 cm diameter with medial deviation of the cerebellar arteries. Scintiscan showed increased uptake on the right side of the posterior fossa.

Operation. Right posterior fossa craniotomy. The intracranial pressure was raised. A bright yellow acoustic nerve tumour projected laterally and medially from the petrous bone for about 3·5 cm and most of it lay in front of the pons. It was soft and semicystic.

The seventh nerve was identified and the tumour tissue removed until only a nubbin remained attached to the facial nerve in the porus. This intrapetrous portion of the tumour was removed at a second operation using the translabyrinthine approach. The facial nerve was densely adherent to the growth, but was preserved.

Follow-up. Postoperatively hydrocephalus developed and a ventriculo-atrial shunt was required.

Microscopical appearances

In part the tumour is formed of compact bundles of elongated cells with oval or fusiform nuclei, but much of it is of the looser-textured type with small oval nuclei distributed in a honeycomb-like matrix. In several places there are large cysts. Blood-vessels whose walls are greatly thickened with hyaline connective tissue are prominent (Plate 56, Fig. 4). Groups of macrophages filled with old blood pigment are found here and there (Plate 56, Fig. 1).

Diagnosis. Schwannoma of acoustic nerve.

Summary

The symptoms and signs left little doubt concerning the diagnosis, which was confirmed angiographically, and at operation. The microscopical appearances are typical with highly cellular masses of tumour arranged in thick bundles with palisading of nuclei (Antoni's type A), alternating with looser-textured sparsely cellular tissue (Antoni B).

While the great majority of intracranial Schwannomas originate on the acoustic nerve, the trigeminal nerve is occasionally affected, and the vagus and glossopharyngeal nerves are very rarely involved.

Plate 56. SCHWANNOMA

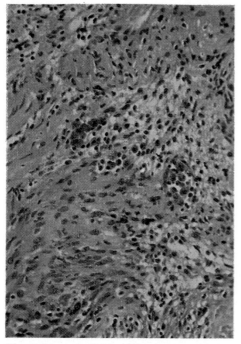

Fig. 1 (Case 44). Clusters of pigment-filled macrophages in Schwannoma. (H & E × 175)

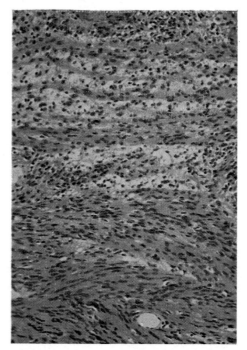

Fig. 2 (Case 44). Compact cellular bundles alternate with looser-textured, semicystic tissue. (H & E × 105)

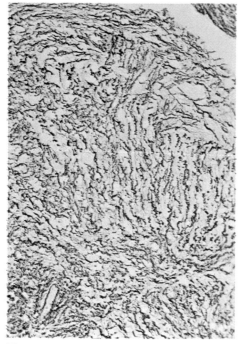

Fig. 3 (Case 44). Abundant fine reticulin fibrils. (Gordon and Sweet's reticulin × 105)

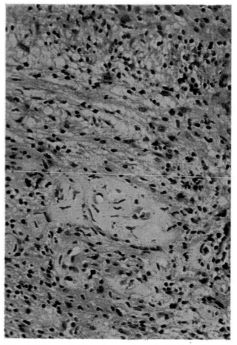

Fig. 4 (Case 44). Blood vessels with thickened walls. (H & E × 175)

SCHWANNOMA
Case 45. Woman aged 75

History. Three years' stiffness, weakness and unsteadiness of both legs. Disability progressed gradually at first; then after an acute episode she could no longer walk unaided. Finally she could not stand. She had urgency of micturition and had been incontinent of urine several times.

Examination. No abnormality in mental functions, cranial nerves or upper limbs. Both legs held in extension with frequent flexor spasms. Slight movement possible at toes; no other voluntary movement. Knee and ankle jerks abnormally brisk and equal; plantar responses extensor. There was a sensory level at D6 below which there was impairment of sensation to pin prick and touch. Vibration sense and position sense reduced at ankles.

Investigations. Cerebrospinal fluid contained no cells. Protein 420 mg/100 ml. Lumbar myelogram showed partial obstruction at D7 by an intradural extramedullary tumour.

Operation. Thoracic laminectomy D4–D8. The arachnoid was greatly thickened. The spinal cord was displaced to the right by an oval yellow-grey tumour 2 × 1·5 cm attached to the left posterior root of D6. The root was clipped and the tumour removed completely.

Follow-up. Slow improvement in function of legs. Two years later was walking with the aid of a frame.

Microscopical appearances

The tumour cells are spindle-shaped with elongated nuclei and are fairly regular in size. Their arrangement varies from compact masses of cells running in criss-crossing bundles to looser textured zones with oedematous stroma (Antoni A and B). There is 'palisading' of nuclei (Plate 57, Fig. 1). The tumour is rich in fine reticulin fibres.

Diagnosis. Schwannoma.

Summary

Schwannoma and meningioma are the two common benign tumours that produce signs of compression of the spinal cord and, according to Slooff, Kernohan and MacCarty (1964), Schwannoma is the commonest spinal tumour (29 per cent of their material). In this case the disease developed insidiously over three years and after removal of the tumour a gradual improvement was obtained.

Plate 57. SCHWANNOMA

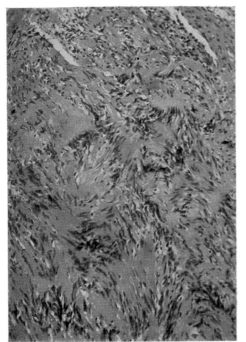

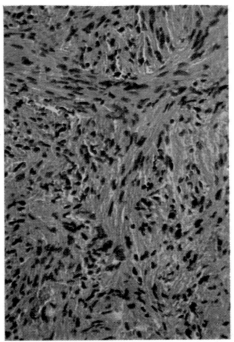

Fig. 1 (Case 45). Interlacing bundles of cells with elongated nuclei showing marked 'palisading'. (H & E   × 105)

Fig. 2 (Case 45). A compact tumour mass. (H & E × 175)

MALIGNANT SCHWANNOMA

Case 46. Man aged 40

History. Multiple neurofibromatosis from birth. Mother also affected. Four months' intermittent ache in the back of the right thigh radiating to the outer side of the right knee and worse at night. Three months' numbness of right buttock. He developed a limp in the right leg.

Examination. Numerous rounded swellings in the skin of the trunk and abdomen and many *café-au-lait* spots. Hearing normal. Wasting of muscles of right thigh and buttock. Weakness of right hamstrings and gastrocnemii. Impaired sensation to pinprick and to light touch over segments S2, 3 and 4. Ankle jerks absent. A hard fixed mass on the posterior pelvic wall was palpable per rectum.

Investigations. Radiographs of spine revealed destruction of most of the sacrum below the first segment suggesting a malignant tumour. Cerebrospinal fluid clear, no cells, protein 140 mg/100 ml. Myelograms showed flattening of the anterior and right side of the theca at S2.

Operation. Sacral laminectomy (S1–S4). Removal of the laminae revealed tumour tissue protruding through the S1 and S2 laminae. A large mass, probably arising from the right S1 root, displacing the theca from S2 level downwards. The sacral roots ran through the tumour tissue, and as it was impossible to remove the growth entirely without damage to the roots only a partial removal was attempted.

Follow-up. Postoperative progress excellent, with improvement of the pain in the right leg, but the sensory loss remained. Ten months later he died from recurrent tumour and cachexia.

Microscopical appearances

The tumour varies from typical benign Schwannoma to sarcoma. In part it is characterized by compact interwoven bundles of long bipolar cells, with pale cytoplasm and oval or rod-shaped nuclei of variable chromatin content, with a little looser-textured semicystic tissue. This type of growth merges with a more densely cellular type, in which oval and spindle-shaped cells with hyperchromatic pleomorphic nuclei are closely packed in broad bundles (Plate 58, Fig. 1) or in large compact masses. Here mitoses are frequent. There is abundant fine reticulin fibre throughout the tumour (Plate 58, Fig. 3).

Diagnosis. Malignant Schwannoma.

Summary

It is very uncommon for Schwannomas or neurofibromas to undergo malignant changes, except (rarely) in cases of neurofibromatosis. The growth in this case formed an extensive mass involving several nerve roots with destruction of the sacrum. A transition was evident, microscopically, from Schwannoma to sarcoma. This has been observed more frequently in peripheral-nerve Schwannomas and metaplasia with the formation of osteoid tissue and cartilage has been reported (Russell and Rubinstein 1971, pp. 293–4).

Plate 58. MALIGNANT SCHWANNOMA

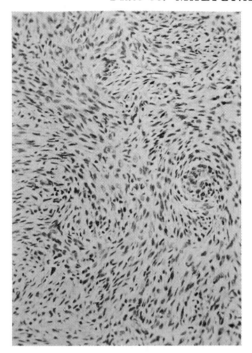

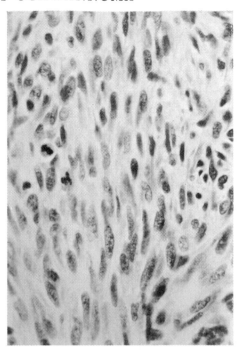

Fig. 1 (Case 46). Densely cellular bundles of tumour. (H & E × 175)

Fig. 2 (Case 46). Hyperchromatic spindle-cells varying in shape and size. Mitotic figures are present. (H & E × 660)

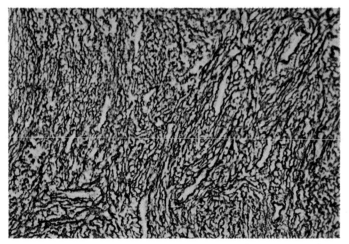

Fig. 3 (Case 46). Abundant fine reticulin. (Reticulin × 175)

Midline tumours of pineal and suprasellar regions

Tumours involving the pineal body are rare. They can be divided into: (*a*) the group of germinal tumours and teratomas, and (*b*) the group of true tumours of the pineal parenchymal cells—pineoblastoma and pineocytoma.

Of all these the commonest is the tumour that has at times been called 'pinealoma' or 'atypical teratoma', but is now generally known as 'germinoma' as this name emphasizes the resemblance with germ-cell tumours of the mediastinum or organs such as the testis. Within the cranium 'germinomas' are also known to arise in other midline situations such as the suprasellar region and here they have often been called, confusingly, 'ectopic pinealomas' (Plate 59, Fig. 3). Dayan et al. (1966) in their report of nine fresh cases listed eighty-seven examples of germinoma, of which seventy-seven were male and ten female. The majority of patients were under twenty-five years of age. The tumours are usually malignant and tend to invade brain substance and to metastasize via the cerebrospinal fluid. Microscopical appearances are of large spheroidal or polyhedral cells with large round vesicular nuclei and clearly defined cell margins, separated into groups by tracts of connective tissue containing numerous lymphocytes. In a few examples this pattern is not well defined and then the tumour may be mistaken for a secondary carcinoma or for a lymphoreticular neoplasm.

The true teratomas present a wide range of appearances. They may contain glandular or squamous epithelium, cartilage and even neuroectodermal tissue. Sometimes they include areas of typical 'germinoma'. Two forms of teratoma deserve special mention: (*a*) chorion-carcinoma: microscopical appearances resemble syncytiotrophoblast and cytotrophoblast with villi and giant cells (Plate 59, Fig. 2); (*b*) embryonal carcinoma, resembling embryonal carcinoma of the testis, in which tall columnar cells and solid sheets of embryonal cells enclosed in a layer of cuboidal cells may be found (Borit 1969).

Tumours of pineal parenchyma may be divided into the pineocytoma composed of relatively mature cells with a tendency to be arranged in small rosettes (Plate 59, Fig. 1) and the pineoblastoma, a tumour of immature cells with a close similarity to the cerebellar medulloblastoma. Gangliogliomatous differentiation in a pineocytoma has been described (Rubinstein and Okazaki 1970).

Bibliography

BORIT, A. (1969) *J. Path.*, **97**, 165 (Embryonal carcinoma).
DAYAN, A. D., MARSHALL, A. H. E., MILLER, A. A., PICK, F. J. and RANKIN, N. E. (1966) *J. Path Bact.*, **92.** 1 (Ten cases of 'germinoma' reported, literature reviewed).
RUBINSTEIN, L. J. and OKAZAKI, H. (1970) *J. Path.*, **102,** 27.
RUSSELL, DOROTHY S. (1944) *J. Path. Bact.*, **56**, 145 (Discusses relationship of 'pinealoma' to teratoma).
RUSSELL, DOROTHY S. and RUBINSTEIN, L. J. (1971) See p. x.
SMITH, R. A., III and ESTRIDGE, M. N. (1974) In *Handbook of Clinical Neurology: Tumours of the Brain and Skull*, ed. P. J. Vinken and G. W. Bruyn, vol. 17, p. 648. Amsterdam: North Holland.
TABUCHI, K., YAMADO, O. and NISHIMOTO, A. (1973) *Acta neuropath.*, **24**, 117 (Ultrastructure).

Plate 59. PINEAL TUMOURS

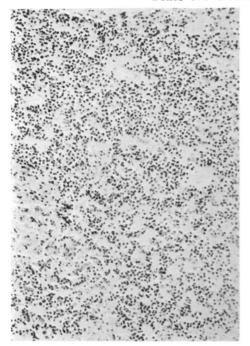

Fig. 1. Pineocytoma. Small cells with spheroidal nuclei arranged in rosettes. (H & E × 175)

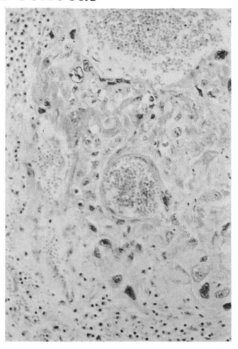

Fig. 2. Chorioncarcinoma of pineal. In this variety of teratoma there is a resemblance to trophoblast. (H & E × 175)

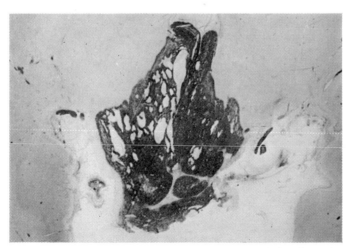

Fig. 3. Germinoma filling the third ventricle and replacing the optic chiasm. (Nissl × 2)

PINEAL TUMOUR
Case 47. Woman aged 26

History. One year's gradual loss of appetite, polydypsia and polyuria. Five months' apathy, loss of interest and progressive drowsiness. Two weeks' rapid deterioration of mental function; sleeping twenty-two hours out of twenty-four. Previously healthy and energetic.

Examination. Confused, disorientated and extremely drowsy. Optic fundi normal. Pupils moderate size, very sluggish reaction to light and accommodation. Reduction of upward conjugate gaze, but other eye movements normal. No nystagmus. Right upper motor neuron facial paresis; all reflexes brisk and plantar responses sometimes extensor; mild left cerebellar ataxia.

Investigations. Ventriculogram showed symmetrical hydrocephalus due to two lesions: a large rounded defect at the anterior end of the third ventricle and the other much smaller in the tectal plate.

Clinical diagnosis. Cystic craniopharyngioma, glioma or pineal tumour were considered.

Operation. Right frontal craniotomy. Right and left optic nerves were broadened. Behind the chiasm blue glistening tumour extended from the sella up to the third ventricle; only small pieces could be removed because of the prefixed chiasm. The ventricles were drained.

At first her condition was satisfactory but then deteriorated, with increasing confusion, bitemporal field defects and a left sixth nerve palsy. It was then decided to try to attempt a more radical removal of the third ventricular tumour and relieve the pressure on the upper midbrain by dividing the tentorium.

Second operation. Right posterior temporal craniotomy. The right leaf of the tentorium was divided up to the hiatus to decompress the brain-stem. The mass of vascular tumour was subtotally removed from under the third ventricle up to the posterior margin of the chiasm.

Follow-up. The operation relieved the hydrocephalus and gradual improvement in mental function followed after a course of radiotherapy. On review three years later she was suffering from some recurrent headaches and difficulty in reading due to persisting bitemporal field defects. Signs: primary optic atrophy; no elevation of the eyes above the horizontal; Argyll-Robertson pupils. Two years later, continued symptomatic improvement. Diabetes insipidus controlled with vasopressin spray.

Microscopical appearances

The two operative specimens contain similar tumour composed of two cell types. There are large polygonal cells with eosinophil cytoplasm, often in mitotic division, and groups of small cells with dark-staining nuclei and little cytoplasm typical of lymphocytes.

Diagnosis. Germinoma.

Summary

This was a reasonably satisfactory outcome in a patient deteriorating rapidly with germinoma in both the tectal plate and the third ventricle–pituitary stalk region, the two most typical situations.

Plate 60. PINEAL TUMOURS

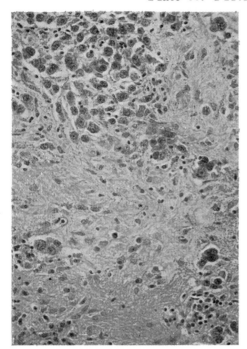

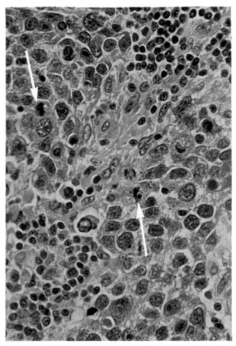

Fig. 1 (Case 47). Extensive necrosis of pineal tumour. (H & E × 210)

Fig. 2 (Case 47). Pineal germinoma composed of cells with large vesicular nuclei and prominent nucleoli, accompanied by lymphocytes. Mitotic figures are present (arrows). (H & E × 530)

PINEAL TUMOUR

Case 48. Youth aged 16

History. One year earlier headache, ataxia and papilloedema. Pineal tumour treated with Torkildsen's operation and radiotherapy elsewhere. Nine months' paraesthesiae in right thigh, at first transient, then persistent. Eight months' pain in the spine in thoracolumbar region occurring in attacks several times a day and awakening him at night. Two months' difficulty using the right leg and foot which became progressively weaker.

Examination. Alert. Pupils: no reaction to light, sluggish reaction to convergence. Left sensory level at umbilicus below which pain and temperature sensation reduced, to a lesser extent light touch. Complete analgesia below L1 segment. Joint position sense in legs normal. Wasting and weakness of right calf and thigh muscles. Right knee and ankle jerks abnormally brisk; right plantar response extensor. Ataxic walking on a wide base.

Clinical diagnosis. Partial Brown–Séquard syndrome at D10. Probably from dissemination of pineal tumour.

Investigations. Carotid angiograms showed no tumour. Lumbar cerebrospinal fluid yellow, 16 cells/mm³, protein 1590 mg/100 ml. Myelogram disclosed total obstruction to upward flow at D10.

Operation. Thoracic laminectomy D9, 10. Opening the dura displayed pinkish-grey tumour 5 cm long overlying the cord mainly on the right side. The growth was freed from the posterior roots. It had indented the cord deeply, but a line of cleavage was obtained and the bulk of it removed.

Follow-up. Two weeks after surgery he was free from pain and some movement had returned to the lower limb. He was given a course of radiotherapy.

Microscopical appearances

The tumour contains groups of large polygonal cells with round vesicular nuclei containing prominent nucleoli and cytoplasm sometimes clear, sometimes granular and eosinophil. In addition there are groups of small cells with round nuclei and little stainable cytoplasm. The reticulin stain demonstrates thick trabeculae of connective tissue (in which the small cells lie), separating the groups of large cells into a definite pattern. Mitotic figures are present among the large cells.

Diagnosis. Germinoma.

Summary

Three months after treatment of a pineal tumour signs of cord involvement began to appear. A mass of tumour in the leptomeninges was found compressing the cord and much of it was removed. Pathological examination confirmed that it was a germinoma.

Plate 61. PINEAL TUMOURS

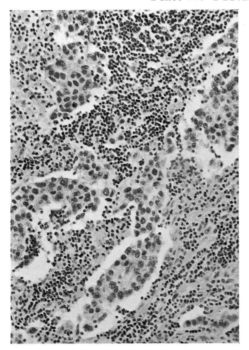

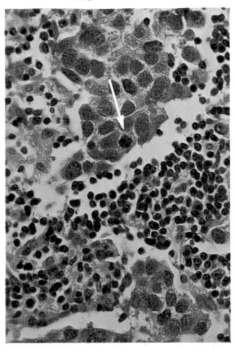

Fig. 1 (Case 48). Large polygonal cells arranged in well defined groups. The small cells are lymphocytes. (H & E × 175)

Fig. 2 (Case 48). The large cells have bulky nuclei with prominent nucleoli. A mitotic figure is present (arrow). (H & E × 420)

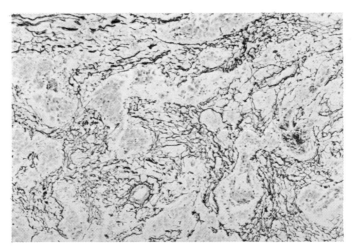

Fig. 3 (Case 48). Trabeculae of connective tissue separating groups of the larger cells. (Gordon & Sweet's reticulin × 105)

Metastatic tumours

Secondary carcinoma and melanoma are common, sarcoma rare. Lymphomas have been considered already (*see* p. 68). Secondary carcinomas probably account for over 20 per cent of tumours in the nervous system (Courville 1950); the much lower figures reported in some series probably reflect the high degree of selectivity inherent in neurosurgical practice. Primary tumours arising in the respiratory tract are the commonest, and made up 54 per cent of Meyer and Reah's (1953) series of 216 cases. Breast, kidney, thyroid and gastrointestinal tract are other common primary sites, and chorioncarcinoma of the uterus deserves special mention despite its rarity.

The brain may contain single or, more frequently, multiple growths of very varied size and general appearances. Often there are small circumscribed deposits at the junction of cortex and white matter (*see* Plate 66, Fig. 1). The cerebellum is a favoured site. In 'carcinomatous meningitis' there is diffuse infiltration of the leptomeninges, usually arising from a small secondary deposit impingeing upon the ependyma or arachnoid; symptoms may be protean.

Bibliography

BARNARD, R. O. and PARSONS, M. (1969) *J. neurol. Sci.*, **8,** 299 (Carcinomatous meningitis; case 61).
CHESTERMAN, F. C. and SEMPLE, R. (1953) *Archs Middx Hosp.*, **3,** 201.
COURVILLE, C. B. (1950) *Pathology of the Central Nervous System*, 3rd ed. Mountain View, Calif.: Pacific Press Publication Association.
FISCHER-WILLIAMS, MARIELLA, BOSANQUET, FRANCES D. and DANIEL, P. M. (1955) *Brain*, **78,** 42 (Carcinomatous meningitis).
MCMENEMEY, W. H. and CUMINGS, J. N. (1959) *J. clin. Path.* **12,** 400 (CSF findings).
MEYER, P. C. and REAH, T. G. (1953) *Br. J. Cancer*, **7,** 438.
RUSSELL, DOROTHY S. and RUBINSTEIN, L. J. (1971) See p. x.
WILLIS, R. A. (1952) *The Spread of Tumours in the Human Body*. London: Butterworths.
WILLIS, R. A. (1960) *Pathology of Tumours*, 3rd ed. London: Butterworths.
WILLIS, R. A. (1971) In *Pathology of the Nervous System*, ed. J. Minckler, vol. 2. New York: McGraw-Hill.

Plate 62. METASTATIC TUMOURS

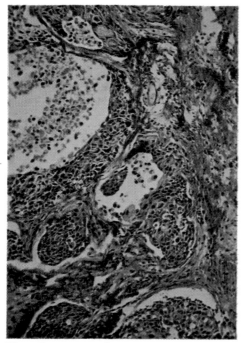

Fig. 1. Squamous carcinoma with keratin formation. The cells lie in connective tissue. (H van Gieson × 175)

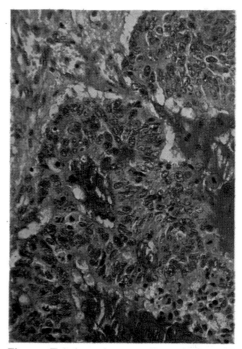

Fig. 2. Tubular columnar cell carcinoma with mucin. (PAS × 265)

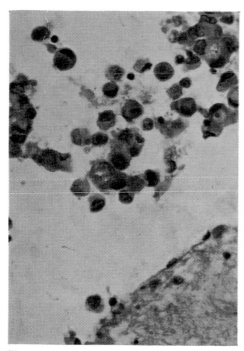

Fig. 3. 'Signet-ring' carcinoma cells in leptomeninges. (Best's mucicarmine × 420)

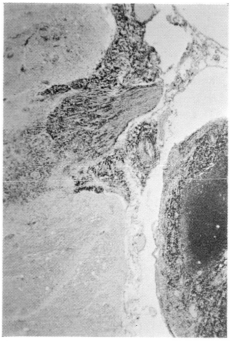

Fig. 4. Metastatic undifferentiated carcinoma in posterior root and posterior root ganglion. (H & E × 105)

METASTATIC TUMOUR

Case 49. Man aged 65

History. (Past) One year earlier keratinizing squamous carcinoma of larynx diagnosed and treated with irradiation. No local recurrence. (Present) For six weeks clumsy and awkward in all movements. Four weeks' increasing difficulty in walking and loss of use of the right arm. He could no longer write clearly and became lethargic.

Examination. Dementia, dysphasia and dyslexia. Orientated but easily confused. Would obey simple commands. Speech slurred. Ataxia on finger-to-nose test. Hypertonicity of all limbs but with limb ataxia of cerebellar type. Stance and gait unsteady.

Investigations. Electroencephalogram suggested a left hemisphere lesion. Left carotid angiogram indicated a large, deep left temporal mass with no abnormal circulation.

Operation. Left temporal burrhole biopsy. A large cyst was encountered and 70 ml of greeny-brown liquid containing solid matter aspirated. Abnormal tissue was removed from the wall of the cyst (immediate smear diagnosis: glioblastoma).

Follow-up. He deteriorated and died six weeks later.

Necropsy. Carcinoma of the left lower lobe of the lung infiltrating the pleura. Secondary carcinoma of left frontal and temporal lobes and cerebellum.

Microscopical appearances

The tumours in the cerebellum, cerebrum and lung present similar appearances. They consist of solid masses of oval or oat-shaped cells with dark-staining nuclei and very little cytoplasm. Where they infiltrate the cerebellum there is destruction of Purkinje cells and granule cells (Plate 63, Figs. 1, 2).

Diagnosis. Metastatic undifferentiated (oat-celled) carcinoma.

Summary

It is a point of interest that this patient, who had been treated for a squamous carcinoma of the larynx, later developed an oat-celled carcinoma of the lower respiratory tract with multiple cerebral metastases.

Cells of this type of neoplasm can readily be mistaken for glioblastoma, especially when there is extensive necrosis and vascular hyperplasia. Metastases composed of small round and oat cells may be mistaken for medulloblastoma and sometimes smear preparations containing normal cerebellar granule cells may be interpreted as 'oat-cell carcinoma'.

Plate 63. METASTATIC TUMOUR

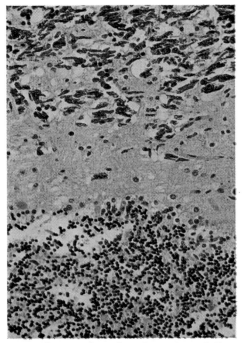

Fig. 1 (Case 49). Oat-cell carcinoma in cerebellum. The tumour cells are larger and less regular in shape than the normal granule cells. (H & E × 175)

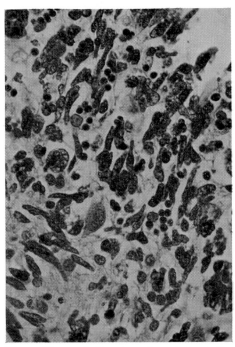

Fig. 2 (Case 49). Invasion of cerebellum. One Purkinje cell and several granule cells remain. (H & E × 420)

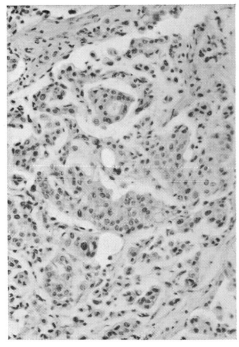

Fig. 3. Metastatic adenocarcinoma of mammary origin. The patient, a woman aged fifty-seven, had a mastectomy four years before she presented with rapidly progressive paraparesis. Lower thoracic laminectomy revealed extradural tumour. (H & E × 175)

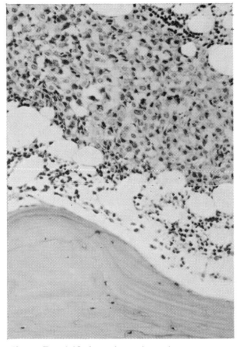

Fig. 4. Decalcified specimen from the same case as Fig. 3, reveals carcinoma in the haemopoietic marrow. (PAS × 175)

METASTATIC TUMOUR
Case 50. Man aged 69

History. Two months' forgetfulness, lack of concentration, difficulty in expressing himself. Three weeks' headaches and occasional vomiting. He locked himself out and could not understand how to use his keys. His writing deteriorated. Two weeks' stiffness and weakness of the right arm and leg.

Examination. Memory poor. Disorientated in space and time. Receptive and expressive dysphasia. Right–left disorientation with features of Gerstmann's syndrome. Right hemiparesis. No papilloedema.

Investigations. Electroencephalograph abnormalities of high voltage delta activity suggested a deep left hemisphere space-occupying lesion. Left carotid angiogram indicated a frontotemporal circumscribed tumour with pathological circulation.

Operation. Left frontotemporal craniotomy. Purple tumour 4 cm in diameter with well-defined edges lay attached to the dura high in the posterior frontal region, with its medial margin 2·5 cm from the midline. The vessels entering the tumour were mainly derived from the middle meningeal artery. The growth was excised complete with adjacent dura.

Follow-up. Neurological signs improved following surgery and only mild dysphasia remained. Intravenous pyelograms demonstrated a left renal tumour and subsequently a clear-cell carcinoma was removed. He was well for two years and then developed *grand mal* fits and right hemiparesis. At second operation a large recurrent tumour (5 cm) covered the motor area and was removed completely with precautions to avoid dissemination of cells. Following a course of radiotherapy the patient returned home.

Microscopical appearances

Much of the growth is of clear-cell type: the cell margins are clear, the nucleus tends to be near one edge and the cytoplasm is 'water-clear' (due to the removal of lipid material during paraffin-wax processing) (Plate 64, Fig. 1). In some places a papillary structure is formed. There are multiple fresh haemorrhages into the tumour substance (Plate 64, Fig. 2).

Diagnosis. Metastatic renal carcinoma.

Summary

A left-sided lesion involving the angular gyrus may produce Gerstmann's syndrome, a combination of right–left disorientation, dysgraphia, dyscalculia and finger agnosia. In this case the tumour was attached to the dura, did not appear to infiltrate the brain and on immediate smear preparations was diagnosed as xanthomatous meningioma. Paraffin wax sections, however, indicated that it was a clear-cell carcinoma of renal origin; the primary growth was revealed and then removed.

While in most series of cerebral metastases carcinomas of the respiratory tract (followed by carcinoma of the breast) form the largest group, renal tumours are also important. Russell and Rubinstein (1971, p. 166) quote one series from Stockholm in which renal and suprarenal carcinomas accounted for the majority.

Plate 64. METASTATIC TUMOUR

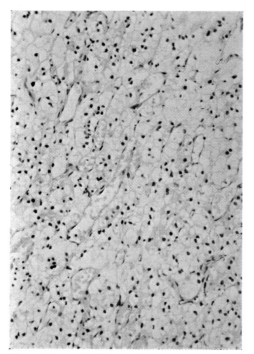

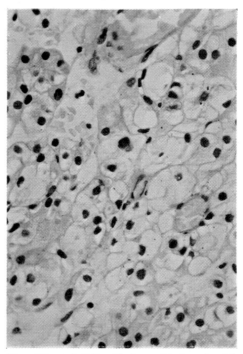

Fig. 1 (Case 50). 'Clear-cell' appearance typical of renal carcinoma. (H & E × 210)

Fig. 2 (Case 50). Cells with clear or faintly eosinophil cytoplasm. (H & E × 265)

METASTATIC TUMOUR

Case 51. Woman aged 68

History. (Past) Attacks of migraine for thirty years. Fourteen years' enlargement of the thyroid gland. Two years' hyperthyroidism treated with radioactive iodine. (Present) Seven weeks' headaches and increasing confusion with deterioration of memory. For two weeks she became increasingly drowsy and took to her bed.

Examination. Dementia, dyspraxia and nominal dysphasia. Could not give her first name or the month of the year or name any simple objects. No papilloedema. Reduction of lateral conjugate movements in both eyes. Right upper motor neuron facial weakness.

Investigations. Electroencephalograph abnormalities suggested a frontal space-occupying lesion. Skull radiograph showed calcification in the posterior fossa. Bilateral carotid angiograms and right vertebral angiogram did not disclose any mass. Ventriculogram revealed symmetrical hydrocephalus of the lateral and third ventricles and kinking of the aqueduct.

Progress. A ventricular drain was established and it was hoped to proceed to posterior fossa exploration, but the patient deteriorated and died.

Necropsy. Calcified dermoid cyst of posterior fossa. Carcinoma of right lobe of thyroid; metastatic carcinoma of lymph nodes, adrenals, uterus and lumbar vertebrae. Carcinomatous meningitis involving cerebrum, brain-stem, spinal cord and many small perivascular seedling deposits in grey and white matter.

Microscopical appearances

There is extensive neoplastic infiltration of the leptomeninges over both cerebral hemispheres, brain-stem and spinal cord, often associated with marked connective tissue proliferation. In places the infiltrate is dense, but elsewhere it forms a coating only two or three cells thick (Plate 65, Fig. 1). There are numerous small deposits in cortex, white matter, brain-stem and cerebellum.

The tumour cells are usually spheroidal or cubical, with eosinophil cytoplasm and large oval nuclei; a few cells have crescentic nuclei placed at the periphery. The incidence of mitotic figures varies up to five per high power field. The arrangement is usually in solid cellular masses; tubule formation is rare (Plate 65, Figs 2, 3).

Diagnosis. Carcinomatous meningitis.

Summary

Two separate pathological processes were found in this case: a midline dermoid cyst in the posterior fossa, probably responsible for the long-standing migrainous headaches, and carcinomatous meningitis from an unsuspected thyroid carcinoma.

Plate 65. METASTATIC TUMOUR

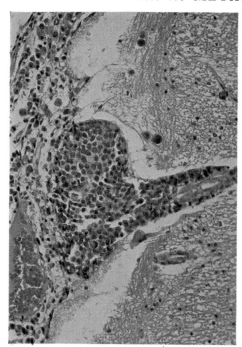

Fig. 1 (Case 51). Carcinomatous meningitis. (H & E × 210)

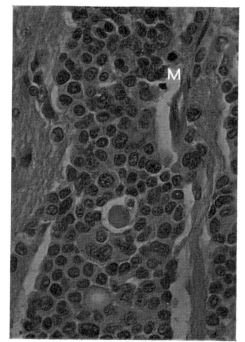

Fig. 2 (Case 51). Polyhedral cells with eosinophil cytoplasm and oval vesicular nuclei containing prominent nucleoli surrounding a tubule containing colloid. Mitotic figures are present (M). (H & E × 530)

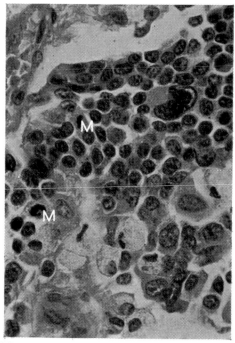

Fig. 3 (Case 51). Binucleate giant cell. Mitotic figures are present (M). (H & E × 685)

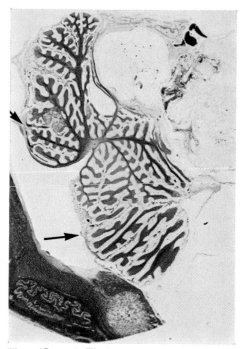

Fig. 4 (Case 51). The large cyst has compressed the posterior part of the vermis cerebelli. Carcinoma cells coat the leptomeninges and ependyma in several places (arrows) and there is a metastasis in the medulla. (Heidenhain's myelin × 1·9)

METASTATIC TUMOUR

Case 52. Man aged 45

History. Two years earlier, melanoma removed from left toe. For some years he had suffered from occipital headaches each lasting two or three days, diagnosed as migraine. Twelve days' bilateral occipital headache and mild photophobia. The pain became persistent and increasingly severe. After two days he developed anorexia and vomiting. Consciousness impaired intermittently. He was admitted to hospital in stupor.

Examination. Slow, but able to understand speech. Disorientated in place and time. No neck stiffness. Left optic disc congested, right normal. No other signs.

Investigations. Electroencephalograph grossly abnormal with diffuse delta activity but with no localizing features. Skull and chest radiographs normal. Ventriculogram revealed a number of irregularities: the body of the right lateral ventricle flattened from the side, the lateral wall of the left ventricle was uneven and the tip of the right temporal horn squeezed and the front of the third ventricle did not fill.

Clinical diagnoses. Multiple metastases.

Progress. The patient died the following day.

Necropsy. Liver enlarged by dark tumour deposits up to 1·5 cm in diameter. Brain: (weight 1750 g) nineteen grey to jet-black tumour deposits were visible on the surface of the cerebral hemispheres. On cutting the brain eighty-eight separate deposits from 1 to 3 cm in diameter were found, some pale grey, some black, in all parts of the cerebrum and cerebellum.

Microscopical appearances

Celloidin-embedded brain slices demonstrate the presence of more small deposits than could be seen with the naked eye (Plate 67, Fig. 1). They are most numerous in the cortex and leptomeninges; the caudate nucleus, putamen, internal capsule and septum pellucidum are also affected, while the white matter is largely spared. The edges of each deposit are sharply demarcated, and there is very little reaction in the surrounding brain tissue. The tumour cells are small and polyhedral, with oval vesicular nuclei; less commonly they are elongated and spindle-shaped and rarely there are giant forms (Plate 67, Fig. 2). Mitotic figures are often plentiful. Sometimes the cells are arranged in small rounded or spherical masses reminiscent of a meningioma, while elsewhere they are in solid sheets. Melanin pigment is very variable in amount.

Diagnosis. Secondary melanoma.

Summary

In view of this patient's history, his rapid deterioration, coupled with ventriculographic evidence of multiple lesions, indicated metastatic melanoma very strongly and no surgical intervention was thought justified.

Melanoma deposits may be darkly pigmented or pale (amelanotic). Diagnostic difficulties may arise when solitary amelanotic growths in the brain mimic a glioma, or infiltration of nerve roots suggests a Schwannoma.

Plate 66. METASTATIC TUMOUR

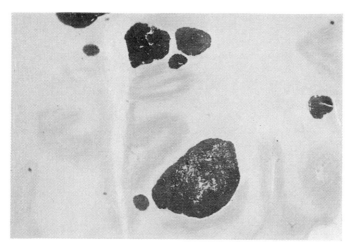

Fig. 1 (Case 52). Distribution of melanoma deposits in brain. (Nissl × 1·8)

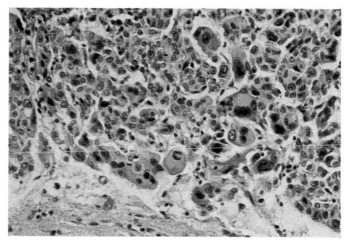

Fig. 2 (Case 52). Giant cells in metastatic melanoma. (H & E × 210)

Rare tumours and allied lesions:
a synopsis

ASTROBLASTOMA

Foci of growth of astroblastic type—perivascular clusters of cells with foot-processes directed toward the vascular walls, but with sparse glial fibres—may be found in glioblastoma, astrocytoma and 'mixed' oligo-astrocytoma. Astroblastoma as a pure tumour type exists, but is of great rarity.

CHORISTOMA

The terms 'granular cell myoblastoma' and 'choristoma' have been used for small well-defined tumours of the neurohypophysis whose cell of origin is believed to be the pituicyte (Burston et al. 1962).

CIRCUMSCRIBED ARACHNOIDAL SARCOMA

See medulloblastoma (p. 60).

GANGLIONEUROMA AND GANGLIOGLIOMA

Tumours of ganglion cells are rare in the central nervous system and, generally, are mixed tumours containing glial elements (ganglioglioma) (*see* p. 62). Small lesions of foci of abnormal neurons may be found, especially in the temporal lobe, that are not truly neoplastic and best regarded as hamartomatous.

GAGEL'S GRANULOMA

Histiocytosis-X involving the hypothalamus (Kepes and Kepes 1969). A tumour-like lesion composed of histiocytes, lymphocytes and eosinophil leucocytes.

GLIOMATOSIS CEREBRI

Extensive diffuse gliomatous overgrowth involving both hemispheres usually of astrocytic type.

GLOMUS JUGULARE TUMOUR OR CHEMODECTOMA

Tumours arising from the chemoreceptor cells adjacent to the jugular bulb may produce neurological symptoms due to involvement of posterior fossa structures.

INFUNDIBULOMA

A name sometimes employed for the pilocytic astrocytoma of the third ventricle.

LIPOMA

Lipomas may be found within the skull and spinal canal and are considered to be of maldevelopmental origin. They tend to involve the corpus callosum. They are rarely found in the cerebellum (Schmid 1973).

MEDULLOEPITHELIOMA

Very rare malignant tumour of cerebral hemispheres in infancy, containing epithelial structures resembling primitive neural tube lying in a stroma rich in connective tissue (Treip 1957; Karch and Urich 1972).

MEDULLOMYOBLASTOMA

A rare variant of medulloblastoma cerebelli containing muscle fibres. It is usually regarded as a form of teratoma.

MONSTROCELLULAR SARCOMA

Malignant neoplasm containing numbers of bizarre giant cells with large single or multiple nuclei, sometimes resembling ganglion cells. Different authorities vary in their interpretation of these appearances; Russell and Rubinstein regard these tumours as glioblastoma.

NEUROEPITHELIOMA

An ill-defined tumour. The majority of cases given this name are probably ependymomas.

NASAL 'GLIOMA'

A heterotopic mass of mature glial tissue found intranasally.

OLFACTORY NEUROBLASTOMA

Tumour derived from the olfactory mucosa which may spread to involve the sinuses, skull, and even the brain. It is composed of mainly undifferentiated cells of neuroblastic type origin: neurofibrils can usually be demonstrated (Hamilton et al. 1973).

PERITHELIAL SARCOMA

Synonym for tumours of lymphoreticular tissue in the nervous system.

POLAR SPONGIOBLASTOMA

A rare type of tumour found in infancy usually located in the region of the third or fourth ventricle, and with a distinctive microscopical appearance of cells with delicate polar processes arranged in a palisade pattern (Russell and Cairns 1947).

Confusion sometimes results from the use of the term polar spongioblastoma for the pilocytic astrocytomas of the brain-stem and cerebellum.

PURKINJEOMA

Maldevelopmental lesion of the cerebellum characterized by great thickening of the folia which contain abnormal neurons and nerve fibres (*see* p. 62).

Bibliography

BURSTON, J., JOHN, R. and SPENCER, H. (1962) *J. Path. Bact.*, **83**, 455.
HAMILTON, ANN E., RUBINSTEIN, L. J. and POOLE, G. J. (1973) *J. Neurosurg.*, **38**, 548.
KARCH, S. B. and URICH, H. (1972) *J. Neuropath. exp. Neurol.*, **31**, 27.
KEPES, J. J. and KEPES, MAGDA (1969) *Acta neuropath.*, **14**, 77.
RUSSELL, DOROTHY S. and CAIRNS, H. (1947) *Archos Histol. norm. patol.*, **3**, 434.
RUSSELL, DOROTHY S. and RUBINSTEIN, L. J. (1971) See p. x.
SCHMID, A. H. (1973) *Acta neuropath.*, **26**, 75.
TREIP, C. S. (1957) *J. Path. Bact.*, **74**, 357.

Cytological methods in central nervous system tumours

While strictly outside the scope of this Atlas, brief mention must be made of certain techniques which have developed in parallel with conventional histological processing. The images obtained by cytological methods almost constitute a different language from that of classical microscopical anatomy. In their interpretation, however, the novice will find knowledge of appearances of routine sections to be an invaluable asset.

Cerebrospinal fluid cytology

The identification of tumour cells in the CSF is of obvious value in diagnosis. In the past difficulties have arisen due to the lack of an efficient means of concentration of the cells, but more recently improvements such as the sedimentation technique, the multiple pore filter ('Millipore') and the cytocentrifuge have enabled satisfactory preparations with good numbers of well-preserved cells to be obtained.

In general, secondary carcinoma and leukaemia involving the subarachnoid space yield the highest recovery rates for 'shed' cells and cases of medulloblastoma are more productive than the astrocytoma group. But cells have been identified from such diverse tumours as pituitary adenoma, meningioma and craniopharyngioma (Rich 1969; McMenemey and Cumings 1959).

Smears and wet films

The advantages of being able to make a microscopical diagnosis of a brain tumour during the operation have been apparent since the time of Cushing. The use of wet films with supravital staining has been satisfactory, but permanent preparations with 1 per cent toluidine blue or haematoxylin–eosin are more popular. Tumours of the glial series are well demonstrated and the details of their nuclei and processes are often beautifully presented. The appearances, to some extent, resemble those of a tissue culture. Firm, stringy tumours such as meningioma are less suitable for smearing, but nevertheless good results are often obtained.

Frozen sections

Frozen sections for rapid diagnosis can be prepared with a freezing microtome or with the cryostat, which has the advantage that the material can then be used for histochemical procedures. Frozen sections tend to give more satisfactory results on pieces of epithelial tumour such as pituitary adenoma or secondary carcinoma than on the glioma group.

Bibliography

MCMENEMEY, W. H. and CUMINGS, J. N. (1959) *J. clin. Path.*, **12**, 400.
RICH, J. R. (1969) *Bull. Los Angeles neurol. Soc.*, **34**, 115.

Plate 67. CYTOLOGICAL METHODS

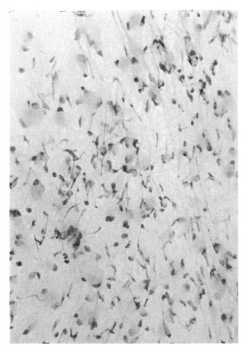

Fig. 1. Smear preparation of an astrocytoma. Gemistocytic astrocytes with eccentric nuclei can be recognized. (H & E   × 210)

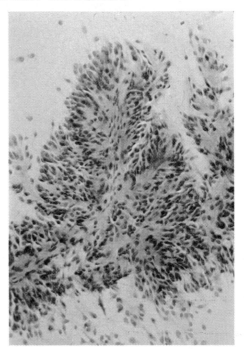

Fig. 2. Smear preparation of ependymoma. The perivascular arrangement of the cells gives rise to a characteristic frond-like pattern resembling a tree or shrub. (Toluidine blue   × 130)

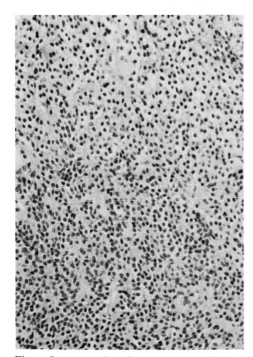

Fig. 3. Cryostat section of a chromophobe adenoma. Cellular detail is comparable with that of a permanent section. (H & E   × 210)

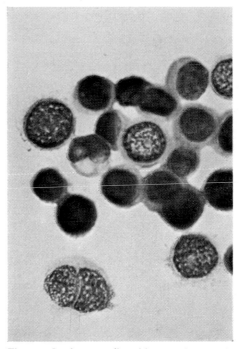

Fig. 4. Carcinoma cells with coarsely granular nuclei and some lymphocytes in a preparation of cerebrospinal fluid. (Giemsa   × 2000)

Notes on technical methods

Fixation of tissues can be achieved by immersion in 10 per cent neutral formalin or formol–saline. For silver impregnation methods formol–ammonium bromide solution is recommended.

Embedding. Paraffin wax is a satisfactory medium for small pieces of tissue and is used for all biopsies. It permits small blocks to be cut at 4–6 μm thickness. For large sections, including whole brain slices, celloidin (nitrocellulose) is used. This method is more time-consuming, but provides excellent results in terms of large sections cut at 20 to 30 μm.

Frozen sections. Fresh tissue may be cut on a cryostat for histochemical enzyme staining and fixed tissue may be cut on a freezing microtome for special metallic techniques and for the demonstration of fat.

Stains

A large battery of stains is available for neuropathological study, but relatively few of these are employed in routine tumour biopsy diagnosis. The list that follows is a personal selection of methods used in this laboratory. For comprehensive information the reader is referred to Drury and Wallington (1967) and Russell (1939).

Haematoxylin and eosin. This general stain, widely used throughout pathological histology, is the basis of most tumour diagnosis. Cell nuclei are blue; cytoplasm and connective tissue shades of pink; red blood corpuscles orange.

Connective tissues

Iron haematoxylin–van Gieson (HVG). This enables the rapid identification of collagenous tissue which stains bright red against a yellow-brown background. Nuclei are black. In addition, it is a useful stain for myelin.

Masson's trichrome is an alternative, preferred in many laboratories.

Reticulin (Gordon and Sweet, or Laidlaw). The basis of these techniques is the combination of ammoniacal silver with reticulin fibres and the reduction of the silver to an opaque compound with 10 per cent formalin. The reticulin fibres appear black.

Neuroglia

Mallory's phosphotungstic–acid haemotoxylin (PTAH). This is the most valuable stain for the identification of fibres in glial tumours, The method must be carefully executed and the haematoxylin solution correctly ripened. Exposure to sunlight or to powerful artificial light sources (such as a projection-microscope) will cause very rapid fading. Neuroglial fibres should stain dark blue; connective tissue tan-brown.

Holzer's crystal violet and Anderson's Victoria blue have little application in tumour work, but are of great value in white matter disorders such as demyelinating diseases, systemic degenerations, etc.

Metallic methods, *see below*.

Neurons and axons

Nissl substance. Cresyl violet and thionin are the most popular dyes used to stain Nissl substance.

Axon methods. These are modified silver methods based on the original Bielschowsky (which itself can be adapted for use on wax-embedded tissues). Glees-Marsland and Holmes are two satisfactory techniques.

Myelin

When studying the extent of a tumour and the oedema it produces in surrounding tissues using large sections, Heidenhain's method for myelin is very valuable (myelin stains dark blue-black). An excellent alternative is luxol fast blue (myelin stains bright blue) which may be combined with Nissl methods (in the Kluver–Barrera method).

Mucins and mucopolysaccharides

Periodic acid–Schiff (PAS). Neutral mucopolysaccharides, mucins and mucoproteins, especially epithelial mucins and glycogen, are stained red-purple or magenta colour.

Alcian blue. Acid mucopolysaccharides (for example those present in cartilage) are stained green-blue. This stain may be combined with HVG.

Pituitary granules

Many techniques are described for the staining of the granulated cells of the anterior pituitary. We have found the combination of PAS and Orange G to be a reliable routine method. The acidophil granules are yellow-orange, the basophils magenta.

Plasma cells

In the Unna–Pappenheim method methyl green pyronin is used. Plasma cells are intensely pyronin-positive.

Melanin

The Masson–Fontana method is used. Melanin granules appear black (impregnated by ammonical silver nitrate).

Metallic impregnations

Cajal's gold sublimate method is generally more successful when used on reactive, rather than neoplastic, astrocytes.

Polak (1966) and Scharenberg and Liss (1969) give details of the modifications of Rio-Hortega's silver carbonate which can be used for the impregnation of astrocytes, oligodendrocytes and microglia. Of these, the 'triple impregnation' is probably the most useful in displaying the fine details of glial tumour cells and their processes.

A useful method for impregnating microglia (based on the Weil–Davenport technique) is given by Marshall (1956). Another method is that of Naoumenko–Feigin (1963).

Bibliography

DRURY, R. A. B. and WALLINGTON, E. A. (1967) *Carleton's Histological Technique*. London: Oxford University Press.
MARSHALL, A. H. E. (1956) *An Outline of the Cytology and Pathology of the Reticular Tissue*. Edinburgh: Oliver & Boyd.
NAOUMENKO, JULIA and FEIGIN, I. (1963) *Acta neuropath.*, **2**, 402.
POLAK, M. (1966). *Blastomas del Sistema Nervioso Central y Periferico*. Buenos Aires: Lopez.
RUSSELL, DOROTHY S. (1939) *Histological Technique for Intracranial Tumours*. London: Oxford University Press.
SCHARENBERG, K. and LISS, L. (1969) *Neuroectodermal Tumors of the Central and Peripheral Nervous System*. Baltimore: Williams & Wilkins.

Postscript

Pathological morphology, therefore, or, as it is sometimes termed, pathological anatomy and histology, furnishes the visual, objective basis for the understanding of diseases. Upon these morphological changes depend the functional disturbances through which disease is recognized during life. They are therefore the basis of symptomatology, upon which the practice of medicine ultimately rests. Wherever a fuller knowledge of morphological or structural changes is still lacking, our ideas of disease remain very incomplete or hazy . . .

Horst Oertel (1927)

INDEX OF AUTHORS

INDEX

Principal references are indicated by bold numerals, illustrations are shown in italics